INVESTIGATION OF VIOLENT AND SUDDEN DEATH

A Manual for Medical Examiners

By

ROBERT C. HENDRIX, M.D.

Professor of Pathology
The University of Michigan
Ann Arbor, Michigan
Deputy Medical Examiner
Washtenaw County, Michigan

CHARLES C THOMAS • PUBLISHER
Springfield • Illinois • U.S.A.

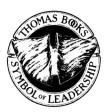

Published and Distributed Throughout the World by

CHARLES C THOMAS • PUBLISHER

Bannerstone House

301-327 East Lawrence Avenue, Springfield, Illinois, U.S.A.

© *1972, by* CHARLES C THOMAS • PUBLISHER

ISBN 0-398-02474-X

Library of Congress Catalog Card Number: 70-190326

*With THOMAS BOOKS careful attention is given to all details of
manufacturing and design. It is the Publisher's desire to present books that are
satisfactory as to their physical qualities and artistic possibilities and
appropriate for their particular use. THOMAS BOOKS will be true to those
laws of quality that assure a good name and good will.*

Printed in the United States of America
RN-1

PREFACE

THIS volume has been prepared to provide information for the physician who serves his community as a part-time medical examiner. As more and more governmental units replace the coroner's office by a medical examiner system, physicians are being invited to apply their knowledge to this form of community service. The professional schools do not present material related to the practicalities of medicolegal investigation. The literature on the subject is widely scattered, and with few exceptions is directed mainly to pathologists.

Dr. Paul W. Gikas has made substantial contributions to the chapter on traffic deaths, and Dr. Edgar Kivela has given invaluable advice for the chapter on poisons and drug abuse.

Doctors A. James French, Murray R. Abell, and R. Craig Barlow have read the manuscript and offered much valuable advice.

Robert C. Hendrix

INTRODUCTION

As the need for scientific methods of investigation of crime becomes more marked, cities, counties, and states are establishing medical examiner systems to provide a scientific basis for the investigation of violent or unexplained deaths, for the purpose of recognizing or eliminating the possibility of homicide. Most of the statutes establishing medical examiners systems are similar to the model medical examiner system proposed by the National Municipal League (1). However, significant differences do exist, and each medical examiner must learn the duties and authority assigned to him by the particular statute of his governmental unit. Wecht et al. (2) have attempted to indicate the statutes of each of the states, but they were unable to consider the special county and municipal ordinances. Furthermore, there is rapid change in legislation in this area.

Circumstances of death which necessitate medicolegal investigation include death by violence, death supposed to be caused by criminal acts, unexpected deaths of persons presumed to be in good health, death of persons who have not had medical attention within specified periods of time, deaths following abortion, deaths of persons in jail, deaths related to industrial hazards, and deaths which pose the question of public health. Some statutes require investigation of many of these situations. Others limit investigation sharply. The trend is toward expansion. This long list can be summarized by stating that medicolegal investigation is required when death is by violence or is of unknown cause. Laws require persons with knowledge of such deaths to notify the medical examiner, and in most instances it is the medical examiner who must decide the need for investigation.

Medicolegal investigation should yield the cause of death (i.e. the diagnosis as usually understood by physicians) and, if due to violence, the manner of death (i.e. homicide, suicide or accident).

PG VIII   —   VIOLENT DEATH IN THE UNITED STATES IN 1967 (3)

Accidents	
Railway	997
Motor vehicle, traffic	51,759
Motor vehicle, nontraffic	1,165
Other road vehicles	288
Water transport	1,545
Aircraft	1,799
Poisoning	4,080
Falls	20,120
Machinery	2,055
Falling objects	1,435
Electricity	992
Fire and explosion	7,423
Firearms	2,896
Aspiration of food	1,607
Aspiration of other objects	373
Drowning	5,724
Complication of treatment and diagnosis	1,530
Suicides	
Poison	
Barbiturates	1,694
Other analgesics and soporifics	995
Other solids and liquids	656
Gas – automobile exhaust	2,049
Other gases	301
Hanging	2,778
Drowning	521
Firearms and explosion	10,550
Cutting and penetrating	521
Jumps from high places	763
Other	601
Homicides	
Poison	60
Firearms and explosion	8,332
Cutting and piercing	2,468
Assault, other	2,165

The determination of the manner of violent death may or may not require nonmedical facts in addition to the usual medical information. Police investigation is one valuable source of these facts.

The medicolegal investigator is not required to perform the police aspects of the investigation, and he should not attempt to do so. Police departments have trained investigators and evidence examiners who have the skill, equipment, and time for detailed study of crime scenes. The medical examiner serves by contributing the necessary *medical* evidence and by documenting evidence in such a way that it can be preserved. The police will quickly lose interest in deaths that are not due to a criminal act; these will make up the largest number of cases to be investigated.

Although effective functioning of the medical examiner system requires cooperation with police and prosecuting attorneys, the medical examiner's office should be completely independent of either. Differences of opinion are bound to arise, and the medical examiner should be free to express unbiased professional opinion without concern for administrative and budgetary problems.

The most recent nationwide statistics on violent deaths are for the year 1967 and are presented here in table form. There are no comparable statistics for the many sudden and unexplained natural deaths that must be investigated to rule out violence. Reports of the experiences of individual medical examiner offices indicate that violent deaths will constitute from one-third to one-half of all necessary investigations.

Since the purpose of this book is to assist the medical examiner in his initial investigation, the duties of medical examiner and pathologist have been assigned to different individuals; it is recognized that in some areas the pathologist will undertake or supervise all of the duties of the medical examiner.

REFERENCES

1. A Model State Medico-Legal Investigative System. New York, the National Municipal League, 1968.
2. Wecht, C. H., Turshen, E. A., Rule, W. R., and Faix, P. A.: The Medico-Legal Autopsy Laws of the Fifty States and the District of Columbia. Washington, D.C., 1965.
3. Vital Statistics of the United States, 1967. Washington, D. C., United States Public Health Services, 1969.

CONTENTS

INVESTIGATION OF VIOLENT AND SUDDEN DEATH

Chapter 1

THE INITIAL INVESTIGATION

THE medical examiner will usually be called to the scene of the death by the police or attending physician, or by ambulance attendants. Any person having knowledge of violent or unexpected death is obligated to call the medical examiner, but few members of the general public are aware of this so they call a physician, the police, or an ambulance company first. The person making first contact with the medical examiner can produce important information. Dates, times, and names of victims and informants will be part of the permanent record to be considered later. In addition to these routine items, significant medical information can be obtained. If notification is from the attending physician, his opinion should be obtained; it may well be decisive. Whenever possible, the attending physician should be identified and consulted. Prolonged and expensive investigation can often be avoided.

INSPECTION

Most laws require the medical examiner to examine the body on the spot where it was found. When a person dies in a hospital as the result of violence or is dead on arrival at an emergency room, the scene will offer little information, but the body must be examined. The site of injury may be remote in time or in space; once the body, living or dead, has been removed, investigation of the scene becomes a police function, but the police need medical advice even then. If the medical examiner is the first to examine the body, he must determine that life is really extinct. Mistakes in this determination have been made with tragic consequences.

As has been stated, thorough investigation of the site is a police function; the medical examiner should not assume this function nor should he interfere with it. He may, however, be able to guide

3

the police examination. The medical examiner's main interest will be in the body; procedures for this examination will be considered later. However, adjacent objects are important; they should be observed — not touched — until police examination is complete. It would be impossible to give a complete list of pertinent objects: weapons, drugs of all types, containers, blood, vomitus, suicide notes, food, apparatus for injection, electrical and heating devices, automobiles, even the atmosphere are but a few objects or substances that may relate to the death. The position of these items, their relationship to the body, and their condition may all be important. The identity, amount, source, and age of prescription drugs can be obtained from the pharmacist who dispensed them and the physician who prescribed them. The opinion of experts such as firearms examiners, questioned document examiners, and toxicologists may be necessary. These are usually police matters, but the medical examiner must correlate such information with his medical observations.

Lack of information concerning the terminal event makes elimination of violence a prime consideration. Careful examination of the body for wounds and of the surroundings for sources of injurious agents will be needed. Small penetrating wounds may not produce much blood. Once in a while, a medical examiner is embarrassed by having an embalmer call his attention to a wound that was overlooked. Injection sites are difficult to see in poor light and are important clues to problems such as diabetes mellitus and drug abuse. Every dead body should be examined without clothing. If any suspicion of a criminal act exists, removal of clothing should be done under supervision of detectives trained in evidence collection.

Livor mortis is a poor indicator of the postmortem interval and will be discussed in the chapter devoted to that subject. Other conclusions can be reached by the observation of livor that are more helpful than determining the time of death. It is necessary to distinguish between bruises and livor; in the former, the blood has escaped from vessels and cannot be pressed out. The discoloration of livor can be decreased by pressure for many hours after its formation, and the intravascular location of the blood causing livor permits it to flow slowly under the influence of gravity to other parts of the body if the position is changed. Paradoxical location of livor will indicate interference with the body between the time of death and the time of examination. Livor will also assume a pattern imposed by the pressure of objects upon which the body is lying (Fig. 1). The color of livor gives some clue to cause of death. The dusky blue of cyanosis suggests anoxia due either to natural causes, such as heart failure or pneumonia, or to violent causes, such as asphyxia. Bright red colors are found following carbon monoxide poisoning, cyanide poisoning, and exposure to cold. A brownish discoloration suggests the presence of methemoglobin produced by certain poisons. Complete absence of livor may, if there are no external wounds, indicate massive internal hemorrhage.

The orifices of the body should be examined for trauma, foreign objects, and abnormal discharges. The eyelids or the lips may close after passage of a small bullet and conceal the wound of

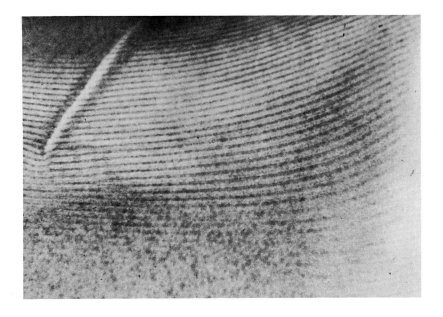

Figure 1. Livor mortis. Pressure has preserved the image of fabric and of a fold in the fabric on the skin surface. It was possible to obliterate the pattern by finger pressure.

entry. An aspirated or forcibly introduced object may be visible in the pharynx. Laceration of tongue may indicate epilepsy. Bleeding from nose or auditory canals indicates the possibility of skull fracture. Hematemesis or hemoptysis to a fatal degree can result from carcinoma with invasion of major blood vessels, chronic peptic ulcer, esophageal varices, or internal injury. The genitalia of both sexes should be examined for injury or recent sexual experience. This examination should include the rectum and anus.

An attempt to determine the time of death should be made, but only very broad limits can be set. Except under very unusual circumstances, attempts at precision will lead to embarrassment and possible miscarriage of justice. The problem is important and will be discussed in a separate chapter.

Identification of the unknown dead is a special problem considered elsewhere. In all cases of violent and sudden death, positive identification is absolutely necessary. The medical examiner must know the identity of the deceased, and he must record the means of identification. Not only must personal identity be established, but, in cases that will go to court, the connection of the body to the crime, identification to the pathologist, and proper identification and transmission of all specimens for examination elsewhere must be flawless.

INTERROGATION

Witnesses to the terminal event can supply valuable information. Their reliability or possible self-interest must be evaluated, of course. Description of the deceased immediately prior to death can often lead to a satisfactory diagnosis and correlation with observable evidence. Relatives and friends can give valuable information as to the state of health of the deceased, even though they may not have witnessed the terminal event. IT IS IN THIS PROCEDURE PARTICULARLY THAT THE MEDICALLY TRAINED INVESTIGATOR OFFERS THE GREATEST SERVICE. HE KNOWS THE SIGNS AND SYMPTOMS OF DISEASE AND CAN TRANSLATE VERBAL INFORMATION INTO ACCURATE DIAGNOSES. Consultation with the attending physician will solve many problems and remove them from the medical examiner's obligation. When a death appears to have been suicidal, some attempt should be made to determine the state of mind of the deceased. Suicide notes when available give important information. Relatives are often reluctant to discuss motives for suicide and may attempt to conceal information or physical evidence. Suicide will be considered at length in a later section.

If there is suspicion of a criminal act, interrogation should be done by a police investigator or a prosecuting attorney.

AUTOPSY

THE MEDICOLEGAL AUTOPSY SHOULD BE DONE ON AN UNEMBALMED BODY. The autopsy and laboratory studies will be discussed in a separate section. There are cases in which absolutely no information is available; in these, the autopsy is the sole means of discovering the cause of death. Most such cases are not of criminal nature. Although an occasional example of concealed trauma may be recognized, the autopsy is not a very good method of initial discovery when death has been due to violence. Detailed, precise, permanently documented descriptions are probably the most important products of the autopsy in such cases. There are many specific questions relating to sudden or violent deaths which can be answered by the autopsy, but it is usually futile to expect the pathologist to determine the manner of death from autopsy evidence alone. As an example, the pathologist can give the detailed description of a bullet wound, but would have no idea how it was inflicted without knowledge of the availability of a gun. The autopsy does provide opportunity for complete leisurely examination of the body and clothing by adequate illumination in orderly surroundings, and with the necessary equipment and supplies for examination and collection of specimens. (This type of inspection, possibly without autopsy, could be utilized more frequently to great advantage.)

There are some deaths which are never adequately explained by the most meticulous investigation of the scene, complete autopsy, and toxicologic and bacteriologic study. It is hoped that criminal causes of death can be eliminated even when no satisfying medical diagnosis is obtained.

Chapter 2

CAUSES OF DEATH

THE medical examiner may expect to encounter all possible causes of death in his practice. The frequency of the several categories differs from that of the general population because of the selection of violent, sudden, and unexpected deaths.

The so-called natural, nonviolent deaths will be the most common; their frequency will vary with socioeconomic situations but will constitute from one-half to three-quarters of medical examiners' cases. They come to the attention of the medical examiner because they are sudden or unexplained. Diagnosis is difficult for this group because external signs are either lacking or are nonspecific, and it may be that the exclusion of violence without arriving at a definite cause of death will be the maximum outcome of the investigation.

Cardiovascular disease, because of the frequency of death without premonitory symptoms, will be common. The subjects are often elderly; the diagnosis should be made with great caution in premenopausal women, but males of any age beyond puberty may be affected. Victims are often obese or have so-called mesomorphic body habitus. External examination will often reveal congestion of the skin of the head and face, cyanosis, and the presence of frothy fluid in the upper airway. These signs are not specific.

Cerebral vascular conditions are somewhat less common generally, and since death is less frequently "instantaneous," they do not come to the attention of the medical examiner in large numbers. Persons who suffer "strokes" while alone may be incapacited and may die before their condition is discovered. There will often be a history of hypertension. The congenital berry aneurysms of cerebral arteries, as well as arteriosclerotic changes, are included with this group. These aneurysms can bleed at any time, often in response to temporary increase in arterial

8

blood pressure. It does not appear that trauma plays any significant role in the rupture of these defects. Intracranial hemorrhage, regardless of cause, appears to have a poorer prognosis in alcoholics. External signs of the cause of death, if any, will be similar to those found in cardiac cases.

Acute infections and inflammatory processes are found in infants, unattended elderly persons, mentally incompetent persons, chronic alcoholics, and drug addicts. The list of possibilities is long and is too well known to require detailed discussion. Important considerations of public health are involved; unfortunately, relatively few medical examiner systems have clear-cut jurisdiction in such cases. The syndrome of sudden unexplained death in infancy is probably infection in certain susceptible infants, although its specific cause is totally unknown. These "crib deaths" should be considered as natural, nonviolent deaths. The diagnosis of suffocation of infants by bedding or clothing requires extraordinarily good evidence, and it usually is not forthcoming. Careful examination of the bodies of these infants is necessary to eliminate the possibility of physical abuse.

Distressing situations sometimes arise when a person with diabetes mellitus is jailed for apparent drunkenness. Death of prisoners should be investigated with great thoroughness, and this particular possibility should be kept in mind.

Most deaths due to violence are accidental (see table in Introduction). The common use of the word "accident" with its fatalistic implications is unfortunate, because most of these "accidents" are the foreseeable results of carelessness, poor judgement, or deliberate risk-taking. The deaths are unintentional (except when related to subconscious suicidal intent) and inadvertent. However, the word accident will continue to be used.

Street and highway vehicular collisions are a common cause of unintentional death. Careful investigation serves several purposes: (1) it provides evidence for possible criminal prosecution, (2) it provides information for safety engineering of vehicles and highways, and (3) it provides data relating to the causes of collisions. Careful investigation of injuries to persons and inspection of vehicles may be the only way to determine positions of persons in the car at the time of impact, or to determine the relative position of pedestrian and automobile. These factors will be important in the detection of criminal and civil liability.

Traffic deaths are often the subject of civil litigation; while accumulation of data for private use by civil litigants or insurance companies is not the basic purpose of the medical examiner system (1), the data collected in the course of routine investigation can be utilized in such actions, and the medicolegal investigator can expect some court cases of this type. Not all traffic deaths are inadvertent. Deliberate homicide by motor vehicle is extremely rare, but attempts to disguise homicide as traffic deaths have been made, and homicides do occur in automobiles. The body that is found dead in an automobile, damaged or not, may be the victim of accident, suicide, homicide, or natural death. The medical examiner should not allow his attention to be diverted from all these possibilities by the presence of the vehicle.

Some single-car, off-the-road crashes are deliberately suicidal. Recognition of this fact requires detailed investigation of the body, the car, the scene, and careful interrogation of witnesses and relatives. The latter may be obstructive rather than helpful. The very fact of obstruction may be informative.

Industrial accidents resulting in fatal physical injuries certainly are within the purview of most medical examiner systems, although the extent of investigation may be sharply limited in some jurisdictions. As with traffic deaths, correlation of the instrumentality and the injury is necessary. Large plants have safety departments which are most cooperative. Small operations may be more difficult to deal with. The broader problem of general industrial health is usually the responsibility of other governmental units, but a medical examiner system can supply information to these units. Medical examiners should be aware of the chief industrial hazards in their area.

There are a number of hazards associated with farming. Dangerous machinery and dangerous animals take a substantial number of lives each year. Poisonous reptiles kill relatively few people; bees and wasps cause more deaths through hypersensitization and anaphylaxis.

Each year, there are about 3000 inadvertent deaths by firearms

(2); these deaths are particularly common in those areas where hunting is popular. All firearms deaths deserve a thorough investigation. Suicidal and homicidal deaths by firearms are also common. Preconceived notions as to the manner of death will block thorough investigation. The deceased may be the victim of his own carelessness or that of some other person. The nature of the wound should be consistent with the situation as to type of gun, distance from gun to target, site of injury, and line of fire. The examiner should have a high index of suspicion when investigating any death by firearms.

Suicidal death leaves the surviving relatives with difficult psychological, social, and economic burdens. The diagnosis should never be made lightly or by exclusion. Positive evidence is necessary. The means of suicide are many and extremely varied in nature. The subject will be considered in detail in Chapter 7.

Homicide is not a common cause of death when compared to others (see table in Introduction), but it is all too common in large metropolitan centers and is part of the daily experience of medical examiners in these areas. Although it is rare in sparsely populated areas, any medical examiner may be faced with the possibility at any time. There will be no medical mystery associated with the vast majority of homicides. The medical examiner's duty will be to document and preserve all of the medical facts and to be prepared to state the cause of death in court as the need arises. Medical examiners do not discover many homicides, but they do eliminate the possibility in many instances. It has been stated that a very large proportion of homicides in this country are unrecognized. It is only by careful attention to apparent natural, suicidal, and "accidental" deaths that these subtle homicides can be brought to light.

REFERENCES

1. Holder, A. F.: Unauthorized autopsies. JAMA, 214:967-968, 1970.
2. Vital Statistics of the United States — 1967.

Chapter 3

RECORDS, EVIDENCE, AND
PUBLIC RELATIONS

CAREFUL, detailed, legible, permanent records of all phases of each investigation are essential. Each medical examiner system should establish a standardized record-keeping system with appropriate forms. The initial investigator should preserve the data needed to support his diagnosis and opinion as to manner and time of death. Questions concerning individual cases may arise years after the death, and no one should rely on memory in matters of this importance.

Medical examiners making the initial examination should file their reports immediately; pathologists should file the reports of the autopsy as soon as possible. Immediate verbal reports can be given to appropriate officials as an aid to investigation, but all data should be permanently recorded as soon as possible.

The medical examiner should start his record keeping at the moment of first notification and should make notes during each phase of investigation. This means that he must be prepared at all times to make written records. The records should show the date and time of notification, and the name of the person or agency making this notification. It should show the location of the body and the time of actual examination of the body. The names of all persons giving information concerning the death should be recorded, and the names of police officers in command of the investigation are also important. Under appropriate circumstances (varying somewhat from state to state), the records of the medical examiner are open to inspection. In some states they are admitted as evidence in court. In addition to the obvious needs of criminal prosecution, attorneys, insurance companies, and workmen's compensation officials will have frequent reference to the files of the medical examiner. It may be expected that some of the persons examining the records will be supporting opinions contrary to that given by the medical examiner and will make careful scrutiny for flaws in the record.

The death certificate is one of the records that the medical examiner must prepare. This document will be an official record of the medical examiner's opinion as to the cause of death, the manner of death, and the time of death. It is a summary of the entire investigation and is a public record. Decisions of financial, social, and legal import are made on the strength of this report. Opinions expressed on the death certificate are not irrevocable, nor are they protected from change by court decision. Death certificates are fairly uniform throughout the country, but each state has its own set of regulations concerning information to be given and methods of filing. The prescribed time of filing may on occasion necessitate making a "diagnosis deferred" report which can later be modified.

In addition to the public and semipublic reports of the professional activities and investigations, each medical examiners system will need some internal reports for justifying expenditures, if for no other purpose. The pathologist will expect written authorization for autopsy. The periodic publication of reports of the activities of the office of the medical examiner may help to convince persons responsible for financial appropriation that the activity is worth supporting.

EVIDENCE AND THE COURTS

The acceptability of evidence is an extremely complex legal problem; few medical examiners will have the necessary legal training to fully appreciate this, and perhaps it is best left to lawyers and the courts. However, the medical examiner must know something about collection, identification, and preservation of physical evidence, such as photographs, bullets from wounds, samples of blood and other tissues and fluids, devices used for administration of drugs, and clothing. An object or substance that is to be used for evidence must be in someone's custody from the time of collection until it is brought into the court room. Each custodian must know when, where, and from whom he obtained it; what happened to it while it was in his custody; and when, where, and to whom he relinquished control. This so-called chain of evidence must be intact. Obviously, the chain will be easier to maintain when only a few persons are involved. Memoranda should be kept by each party of each transfer, and whenever possible, the object should be marked so that it can be definitely identified later. Most police officers are well trained in this regard; the medical examiner should not be impatient with the apparent "red tape." These observations also apply to the body in question. Not only is personal identification necessary, but the chain of evidence from the site of injury to the medical examiner and then to the pathologist must be intact.

Most physicians dislike court appearance for several reasons. It can be time consuming. The courts and attorneys are usually considerate of the physician's time and are willing to make concessions as to advance notice and scheduling of appearances. There are factors beyond any one person's control that make precise scheduling impossible. Actually the fears as to the amount of time to be expended are somewhat exaggerated. Except in large metropolitan areas, few cases investigated by the medical examiner will go to court; only a few of these will require long periods of time on the stand.

Physicians often misinterpret their role as expert witnesses. They are in court to give a medical opinion, give the reasons therefore, and to answer specific questions. They are not there as advocates of either side; unless specifically asked to do so, they are not there for the purpose of instructing the court and jury; and they certainly are not there for the purpose of arguing with counsel.

The discomfort of cross-examination has been overemphasized. If the medical examiner witness is prepared by very careful investigation and careful organization of his testimony, there is unlikely to be much cross-examination. The witness should know what questions are to be asked of him on direct examination, and the attorney should know what the answers will be. This necessitates communication between the attorney and the medical examiner so that no one will be surprised. This is a perfectly ethical procedure as long as the medical examiner does not distort the facts in order to make his testimony fit the theories of the attorney.

Answers to questions should be as short and concise as possible. The expert is not required to give a yes or no answer, nor is he expected to know the answers to any and all questions. The expert is often reluctant to admit that he does not know the answer to a specific question, but if this is the case, he should so state. The witness stand is no place for bluffing; that bluff is sure to be called. A common device of cross-examination of the expert is to persuade him, by gentle flattery, to state more than he actually knows. The witness is seldom cognizant of the plans or needs of opposing counsel; his only recourse is strict accuracy.

The witness should respond without reference to notes as much as possible. However, he should have his original reports available to refresh his mind if necessary. Opposing counsel may ask to see these records; this is no problem as long as they are properly prepared and all the verbal testimony has been consistent with them.

As previously stated, very few of the medical examiner cases will go to court, and the pathologist will probably spend more time on the witness stand then will the medical examiner.

PUBLIC RELATIONS

Most of the investigation conducted by the medical examiner will attract little public attention. A few cases, however, do gain publicity. The news media are anxious to get information to the public, and since there is some competition between various media, haste is important to them. The public should be informed, but not misinformed, and not to the extent that investigation is hindered. Since several agencies are always involved in these notorious situations, it is advisable to have an understanding regarding contacts with news media. The office of the prosecuting attorney is often best prepared to handle this function.

Loose talk and gossip by members of the investigative team should be discouraged. Technical and clerical employees should be warned of the dangers of poorly informed and poorly directed rumor mongering. The results of the medical examiner's investigations may be public property, but the investigation should be conducted in private as far as possible. It may be difficult to exclude the morbidly curious, but it must be done.

Chapter 4

THE AUTOPSY AND LABORATORY STUDY

THE MEDICOLEGAL AUTOPSY SHOULD BE DONE ON AN UNEMBALMED BODY.

Each jurisdiction has its own laws and financial and professional resources which impose limitations on autopsy investigation of violent, sudden, and unexpected death. The present discussion will consider only the ideal medicolegal aspects of the autopsy. Each medical examiner system must establish its own policy based on practical considerations. An autopsy rate of 25 to 50 percent is usually considered adequate. Some rural jurisdictions can be effective with less; those areas which pride themselves on very high autopsy rates are substituting the autopsy for adequate field investigation.

Generally, the autopsy will disclose causes of death that are not apparent on external examination or cannot be determined by other investigative methods; the autopsy will give opportunity for minute examination of the body and clothing; the autopsy will produce detailed, precise, written descriptions of the external and internal features of wounds; the autopsy will make materials available for further examination by serologic, bacteriologic, and toxicologic techniques; the autopsy will recover missiles and foreign objects and relate them to the cause of death; and the autopsy will, hopefully, yield a single, precise diagnosis and exclude other possibilities.

Specifically, an autopsy should be done when it is possible that a criminal charge will result from the death in question. The decision to make a criminal charge is not made by the medical examiner and may not be made for some time after the death is discovered. Some prosecuting attorneys will go to court without autopsy evidence, but this evidence, like all scientific data, is becoming more and more popular. Many traffic deaths lead to

16

criminal charge, so in some jurisdictions the medical examiner system will be expected to provide autopsy data in these cases.

The medical examiner should not release the body of a shooting victim unless he is convinced that he and the police investigators have the experience and knowledge for proper evaluation. If such evaluation will take days to complete — which is entirely possible — it is probably advisable to obtain the autopsy data as part of the investigation.

When absolutely no information is available as to cause of death, an autopsy is justifiable. This is particularly true when the deceased is a stranger to the place in which the body is found. It is also true if the deceased is a recluse or has the reputation for extreme eccentricity. This type of person is often reputed to be a miser and may be the victim of burglary and assault.

Bodies which are markedly decomposed or partly destroyed by fire require complex and technical identification procedures which can best be done in the context of an autopsy.

The medicolegal autopsy should be done in a well-equipped autopsy room by a pathologist with interest and experience in medicolegal autopsies. There has been too much criticism of the medicolegal work done by community hospital pathologists. These physicians are doing most of the medicolegal autopsies, and there is no reason why they cannot make the modest adjustment of point of view from hospital to medicolegal practice. If a medical examiner system can obtain the services of a specially trained forensic pathologist, this should be done, but physicians with this special training are too few in number to be generally available. Abundant literature on forensic pathology is available to the pathologist (1).

A medicolegal autopsy will start with careful external examination, including clothing if present. It may be more appropriate to have the clothing examined by a criminalistics laboratory. If so, examiners from that laboratory should supervise the removal. The external examination of the body requires more emphasis in the medicolegal autopsy than in the usual hospital cases, and findings must be recorded in greater detail. The internal examination should be complete in every case. The brain and internal structure of the skull, the neck organs, thoracic organs, abdominal organs, external and internal genital organs should all be examined. The pathologist who is doing a careful medicolegal autopsy will not stop as soon as he has found a potentially fatal condition; he will complete the autopsy in every detail.

The pathologist should have x-ray equipment available to aid in the location of bullets and other foreign material. The films also serve as permanent documentation.

Toxicologic, serologic, microbiologic, and criminalistic laboratories should all take part in medicolegal investigation. It is not to be expected that all medicolegal examiner systems can maintain these facilities independently, but the facilities should be available and should be used extensively. If there is any question of need of a particular study, material should be preserved until the question is resolved. The medical examiner and the pathologist should know the types of laboratory examinations that are available and should know the type of material needed for each. The laboratories should publish this information and should place it in the hands of all agencies who use their services. The laboratory should be advised of all "clinical" and pathologic evidence. A request for "analysis for poisons" will frustrate the toxicologist and limit the usefullness of his analysis.

Toxicologic, serologic, and microbiologic examination cannot be done (with a few exceptions) on embalmed tissue. Arterial embalming changes color and consistency of tissue, and cavitary embalming performates organs in many places. Competent embalmers do not have difficulty with bodies after careful autopsy. It should be remembered that, in addition to embalming, the body is going to be put in an inaccessible place or perhaps be totally destroyed by fire after funeral services. Therefore, it is mandatory that all necessary specimens be collected at the time of autopsy. The medical examiner seldom has a chance for second-guessing himself. Specimens of tissue, blood, body fluids, and hair are particularly valuable.

REFERENCES

1. Camps, F. E. (Ed.): Gradwohl's Legal Medicine, 2nd ed. Baltimore, Williams and Wilkins, 1968.

Chapter 5

THE TIME OF DEATH —
THE POSTMORTEM INTERVAL

POLICE investigators are interested in the time of death, or the time of injury if the victim did not die immediately. Precise timing of the episode is extremely useful to the police investigator. The time of death is also important in civil matters and must be recorded on the death certificate when known. Medicolegal experts in fiction are able to fix the time of death at a glance with great precision; some police investigators and even some attorneys expect some such ability from ordinary medical examiners. None but the most general statement can be made in the vast majority of cases, and nonmedical evidence, such as dates on newspapers, condition of food in the house, and, of course, statements of witnesses, is often better than medical evidence. Much research has been done, many observations have been made, and many tests have been devised, but there is no reliable method for precise determination. Body temperature, the development and loss of rigor mortis, vascular changes observable in the retina, the development and fixation of livor, and many chemical changes in body fluids have been investigated. These are all changes which are progressive after death but are dependent upon ill-defined and variable factors other than time.

Temperature changes have been studied most carefully. Once the metabolic production of heat ceases and the vital control of the body temperature no longer functions, the heat changes will be those of an inanimate object. The physical aspects of this heat transfer have been studied by actual measurements and by mathematical models (1,2). These investigations have pointed out that a particular body kept under constant external conditions has a definite, individual cooling rate which can be determined by serial temperature readings; thus, a number of temperature determinations at known intervals of time, usually recorded as the difference between body and air temperature or as the percentage of that difference, will determine the slope of a curve indicative of the cooling rate of that particular body under the particular circumstances investigated. By extrapolation, the postmortem interval can be determined with some precision, provided that there are substantial differences between the temperature of the body and the surrounding temperatures, and provided that all conditions such as position of the body, amount of clothing, air temperature, degree of convection, and insolation have been constant from the time of death and during all the measurements. The presumption must also be made that the temperature was near normal at the time of death. Fevers and hypothermia will make all calculations invalid. When external temperatures are at or above normal body temperatures, no effective estimate as to time can be made.

Rigor mortis is stiffening, not contraction, of skeletal muscles that occurs after death. The general rules indicate that rigor begins about four hours after death, progresses to maximum by eight to twelve hours, persists for about four hours, then gradually reduces over about the same span of time. Many factors alter the rate of the development of rigor. It is a chemical change and is hastened by heat, retarded by cold (the increased viscosity of adipose tissue in a cold body should not be mistaken for rigor). Rigor is more marked in muscular individuals and is very weak in infants, the aged, or cachectic persons. Once rigor has ben overcome by forcible movements of joints, it will not return; therefore, the evaluation of rigor in bodies that have been transported is difficult. Rigor mortis, when other factors such as temperature are considered, will permit estimation of the time of death within three or four hours. After rigor has subsided, the time can be estimated (again allowing for all other circumstances) to be in excess of 16 to 20 hours.

Livor mortis is the discoloration of the dependent parts of a dead body due to flow of blood into the venous spaces under the influence of gravity. It becomes apparent about one-half hour after death. The blood remains within vessels and at least part of it remains fluid and can be pressed out of the livid areas; this is not true of a bruise where there is extravasation of blood into the tissues. As time progresses (it is impossible to establish definite figures), the blood becomes at least partially fixed and cannot be pressed out, nor will it drain to other parts of the body if the position is changed. Livor is not a good indicator of the postmortem interval. It is important, however, as has been discussed in Chapter 1.

Chemical substances, electrolytes, and various metabolites and enzymes change concentration and distribution in the fluid compartments after death, and the extent of change is a function of time. Extensive studies have failed to discover any reliably constant correlation. Temperature would seem to have more influence on these changes than time alone. Blood, spinal fluid, and aqueous humor have been investigated.

Autolysis is an enzymatic destruction of tissues which begins at the time of death, or possibly earlier in extremely debilitated persons. Since the early changes involve chiefly the gastrointestinal organs, they are invisible on external examination, but are found almost invariably in gallbladder, pancreas, stomach, and intestine at autopsy. General retardation of autolysis is the result of rapidly decreasing body temperatures such as occurs in death by exposure to low temperatures. Some poisons such as mercury compounds, phenol, and formalin fix tissues with which they come in contact and delay autolysis.

Putrefaction is due to the action of bacteria on dead tissues. The degree of putrefaction is a function of time and temperature. The major source of saprophytic bacteria is the gastrointestinal system, from which they spread through the body. One of the first signs is greenish discoloration of the abdominal wall. Eventually, all the tissues of the body will become dark and soft and distended with gas, and the typical foul odors of putrefaction will develop. Any wound, even a very superficial one, will hasten putrefaction, as will severe local congestion such as occurs in strangulation. Heat will accelerate putrefaction. Eight to ten weeks in warm, wet summer months is enough time for destruction of all soft parts, leaving only a skeleton. Bodies submerged in warm rivers and lakes will develop enough buoyancy by the production of gas to float to the surface in about one week. This is a markedly temperature-dependent reaction. It is said that very cold water, such as the northern lakes or extremely deep lakes, does not permit gas formation and that bodies are seldom recovered from these waters. The chapter on drowning will discuss postmortem changes of submerged bodies in detail.

Insects aid bacteria in destroying dead bodies. Various species of flies find dead bodies very quickly and will lay their eggs. The larvae hatch, pupate, and mature within a few days. Living larvae, pupae, pupa cases, and adult flies can be collected and identified by an entomologist, who can describe their life cycle in enough detail to be of assistance in establishing some limits of the postmortem interval. The flies seek orifices of the body first, and the maggots will be found in the natural orifices and in wounds. A locally dense population of maggots my point to wounds that are difficult to see because of advanced decomposition.

Gastrointestinal contents, when compared with known food intake, may be of assistance in determining the time of death or even identity. Gastrointestinal motility varies greatly from person to person and is also subject to temporary reduction or acceleration. The stomach usually empties itself in about three hours if it is not prevented from doing so. Great excitment, marked fear, and actions of some drugs, severe injury, and death all delay or stop gastric activity. Indigestible particles, such as seeds, further down in the gastrointestinal tract may give some general idea of duration of life after a specific meal. All of these observations should be interpreted with caution, but very important information can be obtained.

The time of survival after an injury (or after a natural catastrophe such as a cerebral hemorrhage or myocardial infarct) may on occasion have some importance. The pathologist can often, by microscopic examination, develop an opinion on this subject. Great precision is not to be expected.

Police (and defense attorneys) often ask about the extent of purposeful activity an injured person could have accomplished between the time of injury and death. The question will arise only when there are no reports from reliable witnesses, and the medical evidence is all that is available. Answers should be given with extreme caution. There are numerous case reports of purposeful activity following injuries that usually would be considered immediately fatal. Many of these reports are of doubtful authenticity, but the issue is too clouded to permit unthinking, dogmatic answers.

In summary, except for some rare, very fortuitous sets of circumstances, exact determinations of the postmortem interval should not be attempted. The time should be expressed as a period with lower and greater limits which will fit the scientific facts and the impressions gained from them. The medical examiner on the witness stand should resist attempts by counsel (on direct- or cross-examination) to pare one-half hour from one end of the period or ten minutes from the other. The opinion should be stated and restated unchanged as many times as the question is asked. The temptation to appear very capable in this field should be resisted. Capable attorneys understand the difficulties, and their attempts to get precise information have some ulterior motive.

REFERENCES

1. Fiddes, F. F., and Patten, T. D.: A percentage method for representing the fall in body temperature after death. J Forensic Med, 5:2-15, 1958.
2. Marshal, T. K., and Hoare, F. E.: The rectal cooling after death and its mathematical expression. J Forensic Sci, 7:56-81, 1962.

Chapter 6

IDENTIFICATION

THE question of the identification of the deceased is intimately related to the problem of the chain of evidence which has been discussed earlier. In criminal cases, it will be necessary to have an unbroken chain of evidence from discovery, on-the-scene investigation, autopsy room, and laboratory to court room. Since every medical examiner's case is potentially criminal in nature, the identification and chain of evidence must be meticulous. The chain of evidence is best preserved by a police officer who was at the initial investigation and who will go to the autopsy room, identify the body to the pathologist, and transport whatever specimens are needed to distant laboratories. On occasion, it may be appropriate for the medical examiner himself to make this identification to the pathologist.

Actual personal identification of deceased individuals goes hand in hand with the chain-of-evidence problem. It might be theoretically possible to maintain criminal action relating to the death of a unknown person, but it would be a difficult practical situation. Often the naming of the deceased may be the most difficult part of an investigation. This could be true even if no criminal act were involved. Visual identification by friends and relatives is relied upon extensively. This may be satisfactory when the death is witnessed or when the body is found in the home or place of business. However, there have been notorious mistakes in visual identification. Deliberate misinformation may be given as well.

Identification by means of personal property can be misleading. Personal papers may be stolen or borrowed. The latter is a rather frequent trick of minors who wish to qualify for the purchase of alcoholic beverages by presenting identification papers of an older person. Confirmation should also be sought. Jewelery and clothing (with laundry marks or store lables) may not be substituted as easily, but the possibility of deliberate misrepresentation must always be considered.

Intact bodies are not always readily identifiable. The ease of transportation brings strangers into every community. The physical characteristics of the deceased should be recorded. Height, weight, hair style, color of hair (save a specimen), color of eyes, complexion, obvious skin lesions, and scars and occupational stigmata should be observed. Tattoos are out of favor in this country at present, but sailors and military personnel who have been in foreign areas often acquire rather distinctive tattoo patterns (Fig. 2). Some of these record names, initials, or identification numbers. Some are characteristic of particular localities. All are indicative to some extent of the personality of the bearer (1). Full-face and profile photographs should always be taken; a good side view of the external ear is very characteristic and cannot readily be disguised; other distinctive features should be recorded photographically. Determination of blood group of the deceased may be of value in identification and, more

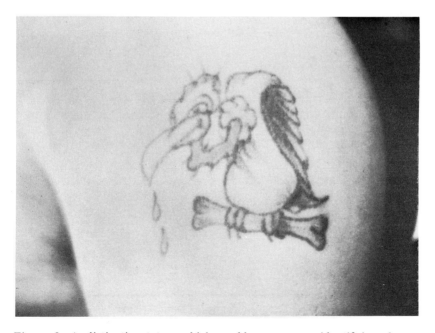

Figure 2. A distinctive tatoo which could serve as an identifying characteristic.

importantly, may permit association between the deceased and blood stains on a weapon, on clothing of the person responsible for injury, or at the scene of injury.

Fingerprints are individual. If fingerprints can be obtained from the body, and if prints are on file, identification can be made quickly. A full set of prints from the body will be necessary for a complete search of police and FBI files. If identity is suspected and only confirmation is needed, prints of a single digit will serve. Some bodies will be so deteriorated that fingerprints seem to be impossible to obtain. The opinion of latent print experts should be sought. All major police agencies maintain latent print laboratories; they can often salvage material from apparently impossible specimens. Most men will have prints on record in connection with military service or employment. All resident aliens and naturalized persons are printed. It is more difficult to obtain prints of women, and it is sometimes necessary to obtain prints from objects in the home of the deceased. This is a police problem, but the medical examiner should be aware of the possibility and the necessity. Hospitals record footprints of newborn infants; most print experts feel that the majority of these prints are useless, but in the case of abandoned infants this source of identifying material can be investigated. It is unlikely that infants born in a hospital will be abandoned.

Thorough examination of teeth by an experienced dentist will give much valuable information (2). Dental work will produce a highly individual combination of details of teeth surfaces and restorative materials (Fig. 3). Teeth and restorative materials are resistant to decay and surprisingly high levels of heat. Even though there has been no restorative dentistry, the arrangement of teeth may be characteristic due to congenital or acquired features. Many identifications are made by this method alone. There must be a starting place for this type of investigation; observations made from the body must be compared with records made during life. It is an invaluable method of confirming presumptive identification and of separating individual bodies in mass disasters. Even if there is absolutely no clue to identity, these records should be made and preserved for future reference if needed. The quality of dental records varies as does everything else, but most dentists will have

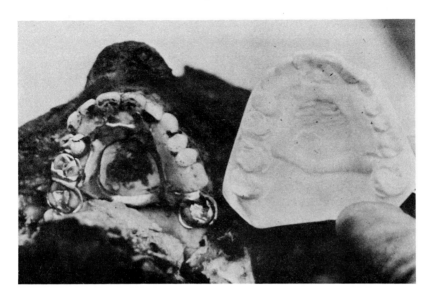

Figure 3. Identification of a partly incinerated body by comparison with a dental impression made before death.

useful records. When possible, the dentist who did the work should be consulted. Neither the medical examiner nor the pathologist has the training and experience necessary for this kind of work.

Obtaining information from skeletal remains (3) requires the services of a skilled anatomist or physical anthropologist. Sex can usually be determined by configuration of the pelvis and the skull, and by the general lightness of the bones. Age can be determined with some precision up to the mid-twenties by examination of teeth, epiphyses, and suture lines of the skull. Examination of the haversian canal system of the long bones can contribute to age estimation (4). Stature can be estimated within broad limits by applications of certain formulae to measurements of the long bones (3). Some idea of extremes of body form can be derived by comparison of length of bones relating to height and width. Race is difficult to determine, partly because of mixtures of races. Skulls that are fully characteristic of Negroid, Caucasoid, or Mongoloid races can be recognized by the physical anthropologist, but many intermediate forms are not characteristic. Congenital and acquired defects of the skeleton can be extremely valuable when compared with medical records of missing persons. Some complicated work has been done in attempting to restore facial characteristics from the skull (3). Although an occasional interesting success has been recorded, the process cannot be considered to be routinely useful.

Mass disasters, such as fires in crowded buildings, natural disasters, and transportation mishaps often result in the loss of many lives. The question of cause and manner of death is usually too obvious to require detailed study, but the identification of the victims will be important and difficult. The need for detailed identification has been questioned, but there are many compelling reasons for it. These have been listed by Brown et al (5): personal feelings of relatives and friends; probation of wills; settling of estates; settling of insurance claims; dissolution of business arrangements, such as partnerships; remarriage of survivors; forestalling fraudulent insurance claims; and circumventing the desire of some persons to disappear and be considered dead.

The Federal Aviation Administration and the Bureau of Aviation Safety of the National Transportation Safety Board have statutory authority over investigation of all aircraft crashes; their authority extends to ordering autopsies on the bodies of any persons killed in such accidents. These agencies prefer to work within the authority of local medical examiners but can override this authority if necessary. They are prepared to assume the costs of the investigation (6,7). The organization of these agencies is such that the medical examiner receives adequate and prompt assistance. The military departments will conduct their own investigations and will not call on civil agencies for assistance. The Bureau of Surface Transportation Safety of the National Transportation Safety Board can offer some assistance with the investigation of mass disasters involving public surface transportation. Local disasters unrelated to transportation remain as local problems. The report of the experiences in identifying victims of the fire on the steamship Noronic in 1949 points up the responsibilities of local authorities (5).

Passenger lists are kept by the airlines and by shiplines for long journeys, but there are no such lists for highway or rail transport and no occupancy lists for buildings that may be the scene of severe fire. Such lists must be developed in some manner before identification can proceed. Reports of a disaster will bring many inquries from friends and relatives concerning persons supposed to be involved. Lists from such sources will be defective both as to omission and erroneous inclusion, but they are starting points. Personal effects at the scene may be of aid in establishing a casualty list even though they cannot be related to a specific body due to the forces of the catastrophe.

The first duty of the authorities will be to remove injured but still living victims. Then the area must be secured to prevent looting and pilfering of personal effects or (strange to say) parts of bodies. If the incident involves aircraft or military personnel on active duty, federal authorities must be notified. Removal of bodies should be systematic; their location should be recorded and their personal effects (if the probable ownership can be recognized) kept with the bodies. These objects are useful for preliminary and provisional identification, but the possibility of inadvertent or deliberate misplacement makes confirmatory evidence necessary.

Bodies must not be released in haste regardless of the pressures applied. Identification must be certain. The process of gathering data and identification of bodies may take days or weeks. In warm weather, storage becomes a problem. Refrigerated trucks or railroad cars can be most useful.

In summary, identification presents two problems. One involves the chain of evidence, the other of actually finding a name for an unrecognized body. The former, while mere routine, must not be neglected. The latter may require the services of many specialists. The two problems may complicate the same case.

REFERENCES

1. Baker, S. P., Robertson, L. S., and Spitz, W. U.: Tattoos, alcohol and violent death. J Forensic Sci, 16:219-225, 1971.
2. Gustafson, G.: Forensic Odontology. New York, American Elsevier, 1966.
3. Krogman, W. M.: The Human Skeleton in Forensic Medicine. Springfield, Thomas, 1962.
4. Ahlquest, J., and Damsten, O.: A modification of Kerley's method for the microscopic determination of age in human bone. J Forensic Sci, 14:205-212, 1969.

5. Brown, T. C., Delaney, R. J., and Robinson, W. L.: Medical identification in the Noronic disaster. JAMA, 148:621-627, 1952.
6. Reals, W. J.: Medical investigation of aviation accidents. Chicago, College of American Pathologists, 1968.
7. Federal Aviation Administration: Aviation Medicine Participation in Air Craft Accident Investigation. Department of Transportation, 1970.

Chapter 7

SUICIDE

Apparent suicide should be investigated as thoroughly as any other death by violence. Some are concealed homicides; some are accidents. The indication of "suicide" on the death certificate has serious social and economic consequences for survivors.

All conceivable means of self-destruction are utilized by persons desirous of taking their own lives. Deaths by firearms, drowning, cutting and stabbing instruments, hanging and strangulation, and poison have been presented in individual chapters. A few highway deaths are suicidal; jumps from high places are also common. Deliberate setting of fire for suicidal purposes seems to be on the increase.

There are several factors to be considered before deciding that a given situation is suicidal. The first of these is intent. Knowledge of the prior emotional status of the subject is important, but it cannot always be obtained. Surviving relatives and friends may be reluctant to discuss these matters. Physicians' records and police records may document previous unsuccessful attempts. Evidence of previous attempts may be present as scars on wrists (Fig. 4), neck, or over the precordium. A suicide note is also an indication of intent. These documents should be treated with the care given to any other form of physical evidence. If the circumstances do not correlate well, all of the evidence should be given careful scrutiny. The special expertise of the document examiner and the latent-print examiner may be needed.

The availability of the means of death must be considered. Persons contemplating suicide often go to some trouble to conceal the cause of death, and surviving relatives and friends may do the same. Eventually, the availability of the instrument or chemicals must be established before determination of suicide can be made with certainty.

31

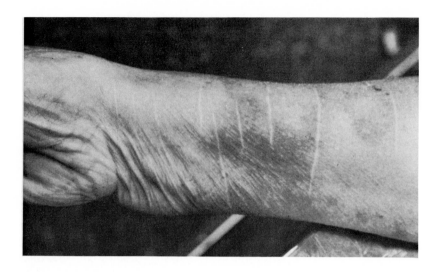

Figure 4. Scars on wrist from prior attempts at suicide. A recent attempt by other means was successful.

The injury must have been of the type that could have been self-inflicted. In the case of chemical injury, this is rarely a problem, but it must be considered for most forms of physical injury. Multiplicity of wounds does not eliminate the possibility of suicide, but always raises the question of attack by another person. In the latter situation, evidences of defensive moves or of a struggle would probably remain. Multiple bullet wounds, stab wounds, cutting wounds, even blunt injury wounds can be inflicted by a person intent on his own destruction, but each and every one of them must be in such a position that it could have been self-inflicted. A bullet wound of entry in the right temple will be a reasonable suicidal wound for a right-handed person, but less reasonable (although not impossible) for a left-handed person. The characteristics of specific injuries which indicate suicide have been discussed in the appropriate chapter. The medical examiner should not permit his attention to be so occupied with the obvious major injuries that more subtle processes are overlooked. The permanent marks made on the neck by hanging (even postmortem hanging) may distract the examiner from the slight marks made by manual strangulation or from injury in other areas.

Chapter 8

DEATHS OF INFANTS

SUDDEN INFANT DEATH SYNDROME (CRIB DEATH)

THE medical examiner will be required to investigate the sudden and unexpected death of infants who were presumably in good health or who, at the worst, had the symptoms of a "head cold." About 15,000 deaths of this type occur in the United States each year. There are variations in the circumstances from case to case, but in general these infants, who are usually less than one-year-old, are found dead in their beds after an apparently uneventful period of sleep. The medical examiner will seldom see the bodies in the original position because of attempts at resuscitation or transportation to a hospital or physician's office. He should attempt to reconstruct the scene as accurately as possible by interrogation of the person who found the body; the importance of the reconstruction will be discussed later.

The medical examiner enters these cases because of the sudden, unexpected, and unexplained nature of the death. The sudden infant death syndrome is thought to be a so-called natural death, although its exact nature is not known. The foremost authorities on the subject believe that the death is a alteration of neuro-cardio-vascular function triggered by viral respiratory infection (1). These deaths occur more frequently in winter months; they are more common in small, possibly premature infants, are somewhat more common in the lower socioeconomic groups, are more common in males, and moderate numbers will have had mild respiratory infections or will have been exposed to these infections. The infants are usually well nourished and apparently well cared for.

There is little that is remarkable to be found by an external examination of these infants. The presence of froth, which may be faintly blood-tinged, in nares and mouth is an indication of pulmonary edema and is found in many anoxic and cardiac deaths. The internal examination adds very little. Pulmonary edema and interstitial pneumonitis of varying, although usually minor, degree and petechial hemorrhages on supradiaphragmatic serosal surfaces are the only findings. This syndrome does not include smothering or mechanical asphyxia. Such deaths do occur; they are very rare and are usually associated with a poorly designed or broken crib (2) which permits its occupant to become trapped in a position that obstructs respiration. Once the body has been removed from its position, the true state of affairs can be determined only by questioning the persons who found the baby, unless some compression marks can be found on the neck or thorax.

The distinction between natural death and suffocation is of greatest importance to the parents. It was once customary to assign all deaths in cribs to smothering in bed clothes or pillows. This designation needlessly accentuated the grief and guilt feelings of the parents. Very definite positive evidence is needed to make a diagnosis of smothering in preference to that of sudden infant death syndrome.

There are other natural diseases which produce sudden death in the period of infancy. Congenital heart disease and bacterial and viral infections are the most common of these. Meningococcic septicemia with the Waterhouse-Friderichsen syndrome is a prime example of fulminant infection. Purulent bronchopneumonitis can develop very rapidly, but seldom really suddenly. The suddenness or unexpected quality of any death depends somewhat on the alertness of the persons caring for the child. Careful tactful interrogation can often produce evidence of preexisting illness.

INFANTICIDE

Unwanted, often illegitimate infants may be killed or may die after abandonment or exposure in the immediate neonatal period. The waste receptacles of motels and hotels are frequent sites of disposal. The newborn is relatively easy to destroy; he can offer no resistance to smothering, strangulation, drowning, stabbing, or exposure. In spite of this, the degree of force used is often greatly in excess of that actually required.

The problem of recognition of homicide by various means is no different in the newborn than in older persons. However, the additional problem of proving independent life processes in the infant is present. The claim that the infant was stillborn will often be made in defense to a charge of homicide. No amount of mutilation of a stillborn infant will result in homicide. The recognition of independent existence can be accomplished in most cases by examination of the lungs. The alveoli expand, at least partially, in utero but are aerated only after birth. This happens very quickly and completely in the healthy infant and is readily recognized even in an infant who dies of central nervous system damage or cardiorespiratory difficulty shortly after delivery. Even partial aeration of the lungs will permit them to float when placed in water. Artifactitious inflation can be induced by positive pressure respiration and by putrefaction. Putrefaction produces obvious changes, and it is unlikely that anyone who cared enough for a baby to attempt resuscitative measures would abandon the body later. The inflation produced by artifical means is irregular with areas of overinflation and underinflation.

Identification of the newborn may be extremely difficult. Location of the body may be the principal clue. The babies that come to the medical examiner's attention usually are born outside of a hospital, so footprints are not available. Blood types may help to confirm other identifying data.

THE BATTERED CHILD

Clincians, social workers, and law enforcement officers have been reluctant to accept the fact that deliberate injury was often inflicted on children by parents or others who were expected to care for them (3). The concept of the battered child is now accepted and recognized. Some of these abuses cause death and therefore come to the attention of the medical examiner. Although courts and social scientists will experience some difficulty in deciding upon punitive or remedial approaches to the perpetrators, the role of the medical examiner is clear; he is faced by a death by violence and must determine the cause and manner of that death. He must form an opinion and must document that opinion in such detail that it can be used as evidence when and if the need arises.

Abuse by neglect results in malnutrition, infection, and infestation by vermin. Often only one of several children in a family will be so injured, indicating that factors other than poor socioeconomic conditions are responsible. It is very difficult to prove homicide by neglect, but some cases have been successfully prosecuted. Many more are known to authorities but without the certainty necessary for criminal or civil actions. A second group is made up of the victim of a single assaultive episode, and the third group is made up of patients who have experienced more than one injurious incident at different periods of time. The multiplicity and temporal separation is made apparent by recognition of contusions of varying age and by the roentgenographic recognition of healing subperiosteal hemorrhage and fractures. It may be possible to obtain information indicating several visits to different physicians or different hospitals. Parents and guardians often present an implausible history of inadvertent injury. The injuries are almost always blunt injuries and made with the open hand or clenched fist or by throwing the child against a fixed object. Rarely an instrument such as strap or paddle may be employed. Burns from scalding, cigarettes, or other hot objects are also observed and may be fatal. The more frequent fatal injuries are to the head and neck. Subdural hematoma, epidural hematomas, and fracture dislocation of cervical vertebrae with injury to the cord are the chief pathologic findings. Intrathoracic and intra-abdominal injuries are less often fatal but are probably more common in clinical experience. External injuries, such as contusions of varying age, and unexplained lacerations should alert the investigating medical examiner to the possibility that he may not be dealing with an ordinary crib death. These signs may be extremely faint, therefore careful examination in good light is mandatory.

It is important for clinicians, social agencies, and law enforcement agencies to work together in investigating nonfatal injuries, in order to prevent a recurrence. The medical examiner can contribute only after death has occurred. His participation may help prevent injuries to other children in the family.

REFERENCES

1. Bergman, A. B., Beckwith, J. B., Ray, C. G. (Ed.): Sudden Infant Death Syndrome: Proceedings of the Second International Conference on Causes of Sudden Deaths in Infants. Seattle, 1969.
2. Blackbourne, B. D.: Crib or coffin. Forensic Sci Gaz, 1:4, 1-3, 1970.
3. Helfer, R. C., and Kempe, C. H.: The Battered Child. Chicago, University of Chicago Press, 1968.

Chapter 9

HEAD INJURIES

THE head seems to bear the brunt of many types of trauma. Many assailants, including those attempting suicide, aim for the head. Its position on a long flexible neck exposes it to accidental injuries. In spite of the fact that the head is well constructed and can absorb a heavy blow without severe effects, head injuries, because of involvement of the brain, lead to death more frequently than injuries of many other regions of the body.

Fatal damage to the brain is possible without external evidence of injury, although there will usually be subgaleal hemorrhage (Fig. 5). It is not the purpose of this manual to describe in detail the patterns of head injury that can be presented to the pathologist (1). However, the medical examiner can and should recognize the broad clinical and pathological categories. An injury that seems minor, causing only brief unconsciousness followed by apparent recovery, can lead to an inexorable chain of events, including ever-deepening coma and death. Contusion of the brain which may produce relatively minor anatomical changes can lead to progressive cerebral edema, increased intracranial pressure, and ischemia. Subdural hemorrhage is of venous origin and presents a clinical picture similar to contusion, except that localizing signs are often present. Fracture of the skull alone is not a satisfactory cause of death without brain damage, intracranial hemorrhage, or massive bleeding into the airway via the nasal sinuses. A fracture line that crosses the course of one of the meningeal arteries will sever that artery and produce a rapidly developing, often rapidly fatal epidural hematoma. Fracture lines entering auditory structures or the accessory nasal sinuses may produce visible hemorrhage; the latter are particularly dangerous because blood may fill the airway in an unconscious person. Fracture of the roof of the orbit or the frontal bone produces palpebral and conjunctival ecchymosis. Extensive fractures, often with comminution and

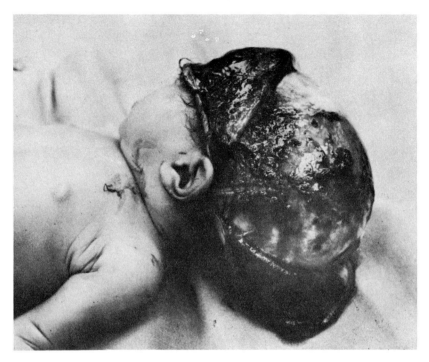

Figure 5. Subgaleal hemorrhage — a "battered child." A very faint bruise was visible externally.

inward displacement of fragments, usually are associated with extensive brain damage and internal or external hemorrhage. The injury may be an open one with exposure or extrusion of brain, or may be closed without full thickness laceration of the scalp. The obvious surface lesions of the head are misleading as often as they are helpful. Extremely severe brain damage may be associated with minimal skin changes; there may be extensive avulsion of soft tissue without important internal effects. Blood from superficial lacerations may fill mouth, nares, and auditory canals, giving the impression of skull fracture.

Fracture and dislocation of the cervical vertebra is not as common a cause of death as is supposed. The marked flaccidity of the neck in the immediate postmortem period is a misleading sign. It does occur in traffic deaths, falls from heights and diving accidents. Death may be immediate or may result from the complications of paralysis. There may be little external evidence of fractured cervical vertebra. The vertebral column may be dislocated at other levels by trauma that produces severe hyperextension. The spinal cord will be transected, and the aorta will also be injured.

REFERENCES

1. Courville, C. D.: Forensic Neuropathology. Mundelein, Illinois, Callaghan & Co., 1964.

Chapter 10

POISONING AND DRUG ABUSE

P OISONING, and the possibility of poisoning, will cause the medical examiner more concern than any other factor. Trauma and the majority of natural diseases produce recognizable morphologic changes, although these may be subtle and require a careful autopsy for their recognition. Many chemical agents have lethal effects without recognizable anatomic alteration.

The vital statistics for 1967 report 4080 deaths by accidental poisoning, 5695 deaths due to suicidal poisoning, and 60 homicides by poisoning. These figures are derived from death certificates and are based on recognition of poisoning by the certifying physician or coroner. The list is undoubtedly incomplete; we may not have even a reasonable approximation of the size of the problem.

Almost any substance can be toxic if administered in the improper amount, or by an improper route, or to a person who has been previously sensitized to it. Even when these bizarre effects of ordinary substances are eliminated, a vast array of toxic substances exists. Just as there are no specific clinical or anatomical changes from most toxic substances, there are no chemical tests which will identify "poison" as such. Analytical toxicologists have a "general unknown" routine which includes analysis for the acid-extractable drugs such as the barbiturates, alkaline-extractable compounds such as the opium derivatives and other alkaloids, and the neutral drugs such as the tranquilizers. The toxicologist can recognoize many other compounds but will need guidance by reports of clinical signs and symptoms, autopsy findings, special occupational hazards, and availability of toxic substances. Officials submitting problems to the toxicologist should collect all possible chemicals, containers, means of injection, vomitus, gastric content, urine, and large amounts of blood and tissue.

Poisons commonly involved in accidental deaths are salicylates, other drugs, and household chemicals, such as cleaning agents, petroleum products, insecticides, and pesticides. Children are the usual victims. Carbon monoxide (automobile exhaust) and barbiturates are the favorite chemicals for ,suicide. Recognition of homicidal poisoning is rare and usually depends upon leads from other than medical sources. One of the important services of medicolegal investigation is the discovery of sources of accidental poisoning and the prevention of further injury

Investigation of possible poisoning must begin at the scene of death or of injury. Therefore, unless the cause of death is perfectly obvious, the initial examination should preserve everything that might relate to ingestion, injection, or inhalation of toxic materials. If the deceased has been removed to a hospital before death was determined, the investigation of the scene will be the responsibility of the police, who will usually appreciate advice as to possible agents. All searches at the scene should be made with the assistance of police officers trained in the discovery, collection, and preservation of evidence. When the dead person is still at the scene, the medical examiner can participate more directly in that phase of the investigation. It should be remembered that several common poisons such as the barbiturates can produce such deep coma that a false impression of death is produced. If the medical examiner is the first physician on the scene, he must be absolutely certain that the injured person is beyond medical aid. If there is any question of this in the minds of the police or the medical examiner, the patient must be transferred to a hospital immediately.

The altered position of the body and its relationship to surrounding objects and materials will be of importance. Convulsions produced by some drugs and anoxia can disturb bedding or furniture, and death may occur, leaving the person in an unusual location or posture. Rigor mortis often develops rapidly following convulsions, and disparity between the known time of death or the body temperature and the degree of rigor is an important clue.

Vomiting can occur in the terminal phase of many forms of illness and can be caused by brain damage. It also results from the gastric irritation produced by many chemicals. The presence of vomitus at the scene should be noted and the material should be saved. Unusual odors and colors are often suggestive of specific agents. Defecation and urination, while frequent terminal events, also suggest the possibility of convulsions. Evidence of vomiting, voiding, and defecation may be found at some distance from the final position of the body; the entire general area should be searched. This is simple when the death has occurred in a residence or reasonably limited area, but it can be difficult under some circumstances.

Some external features of the body will furnish clues to common poisons. The bright pink color of carboxyhemoglobin and that occurring with cyanide poisoning are well known; less well-known is the fact that exposure to low temperatures can produce a similar color. Cyanosis often accompanies rapidly developing heart disease or death by asphyxia; it will also be pronounced when death has been due to central respiratory depression by drugs. Methemoglobin is brownish and produced by chemicals such as nitrobenzenes, chlorates, and acetanilid. The action of corrosives is usually very obvious. Spilled or vomited material will damage lips and other tissues and surrounding objects. Strong alkalis produce a grey, softened area of tissue (full strength hypochlorite bleach will do the same, but requires more time); nitric acid produces a yellow color, sulfuric acid causes carbonization, and phenols produce brown lesions.

Unusual odors of vomitus or of the body should suggest the possibility of poisoning to the medical examiner. Many common poisons have characteristic odors. Alcoholic beverages, phenols, cyanide, chloral hydrate, paraldehyde, carbon tetrachloride, the halogens, and nicotine are readily recognized by their smell. Less well-known, perhaps, are the garlic-like odor of phosphorus and shoe-polish odor of nitrobenzene. Chemical identification is always essential.

The pathologist may discover internal evidence of changes which are more or less specific for certain toxic materials. Even when the external and internal changes of the body are strongly suggestive of specific agents, analytical confirmation must be obtained. The toxicologist will benefit greatly from the information obtained by autopsy, but he will need as much material to work with as possible. Urine, bile, and gastric content may not be obtainable in large amounts at the autopsy, but blood and other tissues are abundant, and there is no reason for the pathologist to send miniscule samples for analysis. Five hundred grams of liver and brain and the equivalent of an entire kidney will be adequate for most purposes. He should be reminded of this as often as necessary by the medical examiner, the toxicologist, and the police investigator.

Objects and materials found at the scene of death or injury should be examined with care. Bottles, tumblers, spoons, paper, and syringes may bear fingerprints which will give helpful information. A latent-print expert should examine these materials first; then they should be submitted for analysis if necessary. Labels, while often helpful, may be misleading. Labeled prescription drugs can be traced with the aid of the pharmacist or the prescribing physician. Stains on bedding, clothing, or furniture may be more suitable for analysis than biologic material from the body. Specimens from the scene of death or from the body should be collected in as large amounts as possible. Fluid and semi-fluid materials should be placed in clean bottles with no preservative. Deterioration during storage and transportation should be prevented by freezing. Soiled fabrics, such as bedding or clothing, can be packaged in plastic bags but should be dried first or frozen to prevent deterioration. Solid dry material can be packaged in bottles, paper bags, or plastic bags, as is appropriate. All containers should be labeled with the date, time, and place of collection; the nature of the material; and the name of the person making the collection and should be sealed to prevent tampering.

Unintentional deaths related directly or indirectly to the misuse of the hallucinogenic, hypnotic, stimulant, and narcotic drugs and other chemical substances such as solvents are on the increase. Indirect trauma due to impairment of physical ability or judgment by drugs is seen most frequently in the use of alcohol; the numerical importance of other depressants, stimulants, and hallucinogens in relation to trauma, particularly traffic "accidents," is not well documented.

Deaths of users of "hard drugs," particularly of those who inject the materials, have been studied by Helpern and associates in New York City (1). They point out that deaths are not necessarily related to doses usually considered excessive; even small amounts may be lethal. This is in part related to adulterants that are almost always found in illicit drugs, partly to the careless methods of administration, and possibly to hypersensitivity.

The analysis of tissues or body fluids for the morphine-like drugs is very difficult. Urine and bile give the most satisfactory results. Liver and kidney can be used if the fluids are not available. Large amounts of tissue or fluids are required. Few of the hallucinogens can be recovered from tissues or fluids. Residues of Cannabis constituents (marijuana) can be recovered from hands and lips by organic solvents such as alcohol, chloroform, and petroleum ether (2). Careful scrutiny of the body for routes of administration and of the surroundings for residual drugs and apparatus for preparation are always essential and may be the only way to explain the death (Fig. 6).

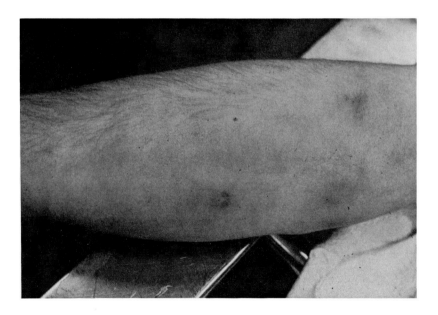

Figure 6. Recent self-inflicted venipuncture wounds. Death was due to injection of heroin.

REFERENCES

1. Helpern, M., Rho, Y. M.: Deaths from narcotics in New York City. Incidence, circumstances and postmortem findings. N Y J Med, 66:2391-2408, 1966.
2. Stone, H. M., and Stevens, H. M.: The detection of Cannabis constituents in the mouth and on the fingers of smokers. J Forensic Sci Soc, 9:31-34, 1969.

Chapter 11

INJURY BY FIREARMS

DEATHS by firearms are common. Guns are a convenient means of suicide, and they are handled frequently enough to produce numerous and important injuries. Bullet wounds are usually obvious; however, some have been overlooked when they penetrate heavy clothing in a partly concealed area. Few wounds can simulate bullet wounds superficially. A blow from a small object such as a spike heel of a women's shoe or the small end of a mechanic's hammer can produce confusing surface wounds.

The diagnosis of death from a bullet wound is seldom difficult, but it is not always easy to decide the manner of death, i.e. accident, homicide, suicide. The decision will involve the determination of gun to target distance, direction of fire, and type of gun involved.

Recovery of the gun, the projectile, or ejected cartridge cases permit the firearms laboratory to recognize class and even individual characteristics of the weapon. In many cases, these items will not be available, and the medical examiner, with the help of the police, must deduct as much of the information as possible from the nature of the wounds. If the bullet can be recovered at autopsy, much valuable information will be gained. A pathologist who is searching for a bullet should use x-ray for location. Lacking this aid he might spend many hours without accomplishing his objective. The x-ray film is also an excellent item of evidence if properly identified. Sharp-tooth steel clamps or forceps should not be used for probing for a bullet or for recovery. If it seems necessary to mark a bullet, the mark should be placed on a surface that has not been marked by the lands and grooves of the gun.

The line of fire can be determined by inspection in most cases. The wounds of entry are characteristic regardless of the type of weapon or projectile. A bullet always stretches and invaginates the skin before penetrating (Fig. 7). There is a moment in time, then, during which the bullet is passing through a tube of skin. The sides, as well as the bottom of the tube are in contact with the bullet. The epidermis in the areas of contact is rubbed off. After the bullet passes through, the skin snaps back to its original position. It now has a hole, often a little smaller than the bullet, which is surrounded by an abrasion collar (Fig. 7). If the path of the bullet was perpendicular to the skin surface, the hole and the abrasion collar will be round and concentric. If the path was at an angle, the hole and the abrasion collar will be eccentric and elliptical (Fig. 8). The degree of eccentricity and the long axis of the ellipse will indicate bullet direction and, roughly, the angle between line of fire and the skin. A bullet from a rifled gun (pistol or rifle) spins on its long axis and bores its way through the skin,

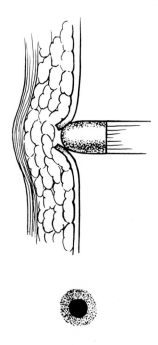

Figure 7. A bullet entering skin. The invagination of epidermis and the characteristic abrasion collar are diagrammed.

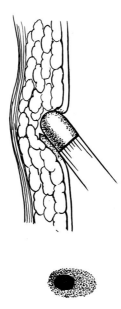

Figure 8. An oblique entrance wound. The eccentricity and elliptical shape of the wound and the abrasion collar are diagrammed.

producing a neat hole. Shot from a shotgun do not have this boring action, but since they are spherical they also make a neat entry. Irregular entry wounds can be produced by high-powered guns close to or in contact with tissues (Figs. 9, 10). There is a variable amount of "blow back" by the gases of explosion and by reflection of the bullet's energy from underlying tissues. The "blow back" can cause a wound that is much larger than the projectile and which can be very irregular; tissue actually may protrude from the wound, but the abrasion collar will be present, and the wound of entrance can be recognized by it (Fig. 10). Skin may be forced against the gun muzzle in contact and thus be marked by it (Figs. 11 and 12).

The exit wound can be of any size or shape. Tumbling, fragmentation or deformation of the bullet, and the presence of secondary missiles such as pieces of bone all contribute to this variability. Since this is a "blow out" type of wound, the margins, regardless of shape, will be sharp (Figs. 13 and 14). There will be

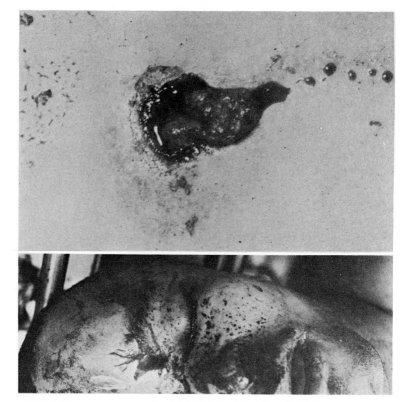

Figure 9 (left). An entrance wound. An abrasion collar is visible at the lower part of the wound. The "blow back" effect is seen superiorly. The minute abrasions on cheek, nose, and eyelid were caused by grains of unburned gun powder.

Figure 10 (right). Tissue protrudes from an entry wound made by a .410-guage shot-gun. Note the abrasion collar.

no abrasion collar. If the only wound on the head appears to be an exit wound, entrance may be through the mouth. If an exit wound is made when the skin is pressed against a firm surface, the crushing effect can produce a wound that is almost indistinguishable from an entrance wound.

Powerful weapons, such as the ordinary "deer rifle" or large-gauge shotguns, can produce massive tissue destruction at short range. The great energy released by these high-velocity

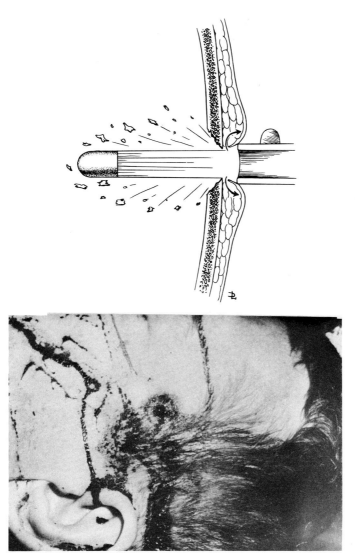

Figure 11 (upper). A contact wound. The arrows indicate the reflection of force from underlying bone. The skin will be torn irregularly and may be marked by the muzzle of the gun. The funnel shape of the wound in the skull is characteristic.

Figure 12 (lower). A contact wound. The size and shape of the muzzle of the gun are imprinted on the skin.

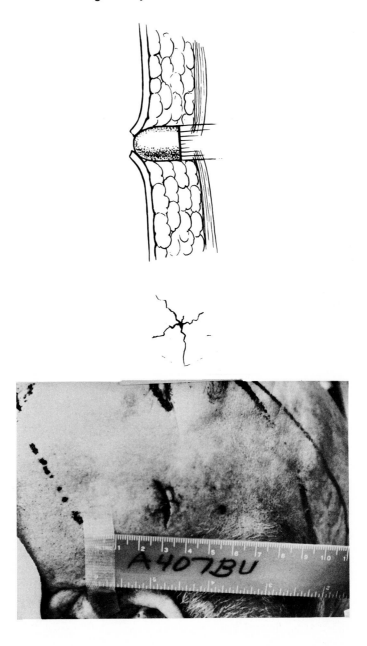

Figure 13 (upper). The formation of an exit wound. The superficial epidermis is not touched or abraded by the bullet.

Figure 14 (lower). An exit wound. Hand loaded, .45-cal target ammunition.

missiles produces a splash effect that involves large volumes of tissue. The wound of exit may be lost in the extensive destruction, but there will always be remnants of the entrance wound with its abrasion collar. This type of wound does not prove that the muzzle of the gun was in tight contact with the tissue. The expanding gases of the explosion are destructive, of course, but the high energy of the bullet is capable of great damage, even though the force of the expanding gases has been dissipated in a space between the muzzle and the target.

Most shotgun shells contain many projectiles and plastic or fiber "wads" which keep shot and gunpowder in place. At close range, the shot and wads are in a compact group and produce a single hole (Fig. 10), leaving no surface indication of the many separate particles that produced the wound. At a greater distance from the muzzle, the wads fall away and the shots spread to produce the "pattern." The extent of this spread is a function of the distance from the muzzle, type of muzzle, the original packaging of the shot in the shell, and the velocity imparted to the shot by the powder charge. The distance from shotgun to target can be determined with fair accuracy by firing the same type of ammunition from the gun in question at known distances and noting the spread or pattern of the shot. Shotguns can be loaded with a single, solid projectile. This missile lacks the velocity and accuracy of a rifle bullet, but its relatively great weight gives it a destructive potential.

All firearms discharge, along with the bullet, a mixture of flame, hot gas, smoke, and partly burned powder grains (Figs. 9 and 15). The flame can singe hair and clothing, however, the "powder burns" are not due to heat but to deposition of smoke and powder residues. If the muzzle is in contact with the skin, all of these waste products will enter the wound, and the surrounding skin will be clean. The gases containing carbon monoxide may enter the tissues in quantities large enough to be detected chemically or visually. The effects of the heat do not extend far beyond the gun. Smoke which is easily wiped away (too easily in some instances) travels a little further, and particulate matter, such as unburned powder and metal particles, travels even further. These particles may penetrate skin and produce minute abrasions (Fig. 9).

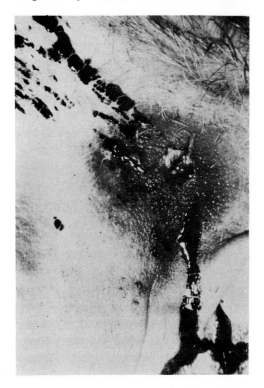

Figure 15. Carbon deposited on skin around an entry wound.

Moderately precise measurements of the gun to target distance can be achieved by firing the particular weapon with similar ammunition against a white target.

The matter of distance is important. Without some mechanical device, any gun will deposit powder residues on or in the tissues or clothing of a person who shoots himself, whether accidentially or deliberately, unless some object has been placed between the gun and the target. The stories of witnesses may be substantiated or proven to be false by this determination.

If the entry wound is through clothing, powder residues will be on the fabric. This should be removed and examined in a criminalistics laboratory. When clothing is removed from a shooting victim, care should be taken not to lose bullets which may have passed through the body and lie free inside the clothing.

The bullet track within the body can indicate the direction of passage, particularly through bone. The diameter of the bullet track through bone increases in the direction of travel of the bullet (Fig. 11). A funnel-shaped hole is produced, with the narrow part of the funnel pointing toward the gun. This is best seen in flat bones of the skull but may be recognized elsewhere. Bullets do not always move in a straight line in the body, but deflection will usually be obvious. Ricochet from bone is possible, and even soft tissues can alter the course of the bullet to some extent. The medical examiner will often be asked to state with some precision the direction of motion of the bullet. This can be done, but it can be done only in reference to the body, unless complete information as to the shooting incident is available. As an example, one may report that a bullet that passed through the body traveled in a perfectly horizontal plane. This would be true only if the body were in an erect posture at the time it was struck by the bullet.

The size of a bullet wound is not a good indication of the size of the bullet. The reasons for the lack of correlation have been presented. A bullet is not like a drill. In soft tissue and bone the splash effect will always produce defects larger than the missile, but the skin wounds are totally unreliable. Even the distinction between large and small calibers is not reliable (Fig. 16).

Few medical examiners and pathologists are experts in firearms investigation, and they should not attempt it. Criminalistics laboratories have equipment and staff for this kind of work. Medical investigators should confine their investigations to the human body. The medical examiner should not pick up guns found at the scene; he might shoot himself or another person, and he will almost certainly obscure fingerprints on the gun.

Recovered bullets can be compared with test-fired bullets from specific guns, and identification can often be made. Persons recovering bullets should handle them with great care. Most are made of soft metal and are easily marred. Projectiles from shotguns do not acquire specific characteristics upon firing, although the cases do. The removed shot can be useful; the size, number, nature of metalic alloy, and particularly the size and construction of the wad can point to ammunition of particular type and manufacturer and to the gauge (caliber) of the gun.

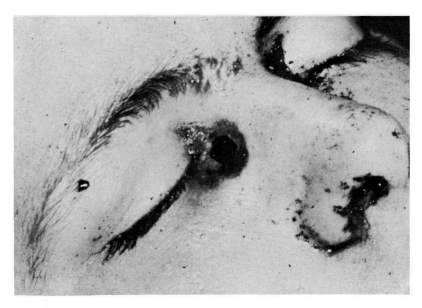

Figure 16. An entrance wound with a wide abrasion collar. The hole was about one-half inch in diameter; it was made by a .22-cal bullet. Size of projectile cannot be determined with certainty.

Certain types of guns eject the cartridge case after firing; these cases may be found at the scene. The recovery is not the duty of the medical examiner, but he should be aware of their importance. The trajectory of ejected cases is relatively constant for each type of gun so the position of the gun at the time of firing can be estimated. The decision as to manner of death by bullet wound may be made in this manner. In addition, these ejected cases will carry both class and individual characteristics of the gun from which they were fired. As the firing pin strikes the primer, as the case is forced against the face of the breech block, and as the ejection mechanism grasps the cartridge, marks are made which can be recognizably reproduced by subsequent firing of the same gun. The ejected cases may bear fingerprints. Only the results of these observations can concern the medical examiner.

In summary, wounds by firearms have characteristics which give evidence of the direction of fire, possibly target to gun distance, and often the type and size of ammunition of weapon. Recovery of projectiles enhances the value of all these determinations, but much can be learned by careful examination of external and internal features of bullet wounds.

Bombs injure in several ways. They may be so constructed that fragments become high-speed missiles and act much like large, irregular bullets with an erratic course. Materials adjacent to the explosion may also be fragmented and act as missiles. Recovery of foreign objects from victims of bombing is important; explosion experts may be able to use them in characterizing the device. Bombs can cause collapse of buildings and produce injury and death by crushing. The sharp wave of great increase, then decrease in atmospheric pressure also produces fatal injuries. The damage to the body is produced at points of marked change in density, so the lungs and the air-containing gastroinestinal tract are frequent points of contusions or lacerations. If the explosion is powerful and is close to the body, extreme destruction will occur. The effects of incendiary bombs are thermal for the most part.

Chapter 12

INJURY BY SHARP INSTRUMENTS

A STABBING wound is produced by an instrument which has a sharp point; it may or may not have a cutting edge as well. Most knives have a point and one or two sharp edges. Instruments such as icepicks — which are no longer very common, skewers, and stilettos have round or square cross-sections and do not have cutting edges.

The purely stabbing instruments produce small wounds which may have superficial resemblance to bullet wounds. They are not nearly as destructive to tissues as are bullets, and the internal features are different. The stab wound that ends blindly can certainly be distinguished from a bullet wound by absence of the bullet; a through-and-through wound may cause concern, but the small amount of tissue damage caused by the stab wound will be apparent.

The elasticity of the skin distorts the size and shape of the stab wound more than it does a bullet wound (Fig. 17). The flexible body wall may give under the force of the blow and thereby allow the instrument to produce a wound that is deeper than the blade is long. For these reasons, the medical examiner should entertain many reservations when attempting to visualize the shape of the weapon from the nature of the wound. Knives, when used for stabbing, will cut, as well as penetrate, and may produce a wound that is longer than the knife is broad. If the investigator can determine that a given wound was perpendicular to the skin, and if he can compensate for the distortion produced by the elasticity of the skin, he may be able to state the maximum possible width of the blade. Double-edged knives are not common; stab wounds made by such a knife may be identifiable by the evidence of cutting at both ends.

Sharp knives, razors, and fragments of glass can be used as cutting instruments producing an elongated wound with very

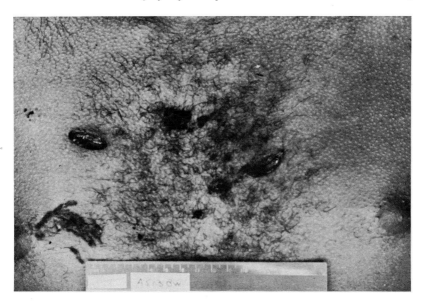

Figure 17. Gaping knife wounds. The length of these wounds closely approximates the width of the blade, but this is not always the case.

sharp margins. There will be little damage to nearby tissues. Death from stabbing and cutting is by external or internal exsanguination as a rule. Direct wounds of the central nervous system may destroy important structures without extensive hemorrhage. Division of the major veins, as in the neck, permits the entrance of air, and death may be due to air embolism.

Certain characteristics of cutting and stabbing wounds seem indicative of suicide, others suggest homicide. The wounds may be multiple in either case. The person attempting suicide will often make tentative wounds with so-called hesitation marks. He may make several of these on one part of the body then transfer his attention to another area (Fig. 4). Several stab wounds may be found over the precordial area. They are seldom made through clothing, which often will be unbuttoned or pulled away. The person attempting to cut his own throat will often make several tentative cuts on the side of the neck away from the hand holding the knife. The final cut may be very deep and end in a single slash towards the hand with the weapon. These wounds often start high on the neck and become transverse as they cross the midline. It is important to know the handedness of the victim.

The individual attempting suicide by stabbing and cutting will often attack himself with great ferocity and do so much damage that the investigator must doubt that it could all be self-inflicted. The multiple wounds will all be in areas within reach and the surroundings will not show the disarray and blood spattering that would be expected as the result of homicidal attack.

A planned homicidal assault upon an unsuspecting victim may result in a knife wound in the back, in the anterior part of the chest, or a cut throat. These wounds are single and purposeful. Most homicidal attacks with sharp instruments are not planned but are the results of an altercation. They are often multiple. The hands and the arms of the victim are cut because they are held up in defense. Clothing is cut and the surroundings show evidence of the fray.

Small stab wounds that penetrate skin and subcutaneum obliquely do not produce large amounts of blood. Internal hemorrhage may be abundant, but the injured individual may not be aware of the seriousness of his wound, and it is possible for him to be active for several hours before death.

Axes, cleavers, and heavy knives like machetes have cutting edges, but their great weight produces crushing injury to bone and deeper tissues. In this way, the wounds resemble those produced by blunt instruments. The general type of weapon can often be recognized from the wound. Even these awkward tools can be used suicidally, and multiple blows can be self-inflicted. They are always in accessible areas and usually produce parallel wounds. The surroundings are remarkably undisturbed in contrast to the ferocity of the attack on the person.

When the circumstances suggest — as is often the case in homicidal stabbing and cutting — that the assailant may have been spattered with blood, samples of the victim's blood should be tested for blood type for possible comparison later.

Chapter 13

INJURY BY BLUNT OBJECTS

INJURIES such as contusions, abrasions, and lacerations are produced by blunt trauma which may be direct blows, torsion, scrapes, or explosive forces.

Abrasions are external injuries produced by sliding contact between the body and a rough surface. A rope burn is an example, as is the scraping of skin which occurs when a body slides along the road surface after ejection from a car. The abrasion is a more or less uniform removal of upper layers of skin over fairly broad areas. Some superficial gouges may also be present. These wounds bleed very little, but can produce moderate amounts of serum. They dry shortly after death and present a brownish, paper-like surface. It is often possible to retrieve fragments of the abrading material from the wounds. At the margins of the wound, epidermis may be displaced in a manner that indicates the relative direction of the sliding force. On occasion, abrasions can occur without such sliding effect. The scalp coming in contact with street or sidewalk may slide very little, but the epidermis will be crushed and resemble an abrasion. A blow from a rough-textured, flat object may have the same effect. If the abrading surface has a pattern and there is not too much sliding, the pattern will be impressed on the skin (Figs. 18 and 19). The threaded ends of a pipe, the ribbed surface of some varieties of garden hose, and the treads of tires produce identifiable patterns of abrasions. Abrasions are not fatal or even very serious injuries, but the force which produced them may have produced more extensive damage.

A contusion or bruise results from traumatic damage to tissue, with rupture of capillaries. Epidermis over a cutaneous contusion may or may not be abraded. Bleeding associated with some vascular diseases and hemorrhagic diatheses occurs with such slight trauma that it is often called "spontaneous" hemorrhage. The underlying disease outweighs the hemorrhage in importance. Brief

61

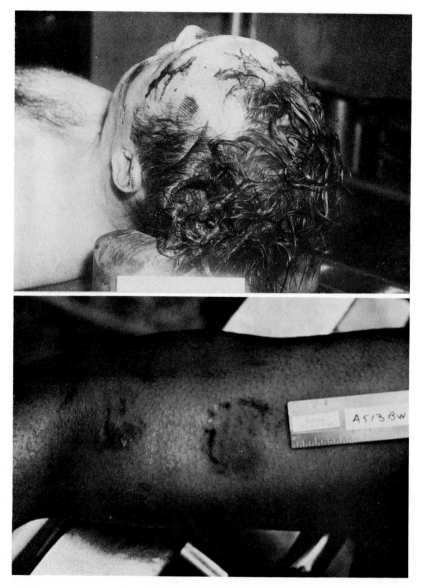

Figure 18 (upper). Patterned abrasions. Pipe threads. Homicide.

Figure 19 (lower). Human bite. Misalignment of teeth may be characteristic and may permit identification of the "weapon." The scars in the antecubital fossa are from self-injection of drugs.

study should indicate the basically nontraumatic nature of these conditions.

Contusions occur only during life. Damage to blood vessels after death produces some extravasation of blood but not into tissues. Contusions must be differentiated from the much more common livor mortis. The blood producing the discoloration of a contusion is extravascular and cannot be pressed out of the tissues. The bruise may or may not be swollen. It will be reddish blue when first formed, then darker blue. Over a period of days, with the breakdown of hemoglobin, the color will change to green, brown, and then yellow. The latter color may be visible for a long time, and microscopic evidence may persist for years. This change in color can be used in a rough way to determine time of survival after injury. It is particularly important to note bruises of different ages indicating several episodes of trauma. This type of evidence is often the first cause of suspicion in dealing with battered children. Parents will report a single, implausible traumatic episode, and examination will show that there have been repeated episodes. Extravasation of blood into the soft tissue of the upper eyelid often follows direct trauma. This is the ordinary black eye. This appearance can also follow fracture of the anterior portion of the skull and may not indicate direct trauma to the orbital area. Every tissue can be bruised, regardless of its location in the body. Most of these are relatively inocuous. Exceptions are the contusions of the brain (which have been considered in Chapter 9) and of the heart, both of which can be fatal. Blunt injury to the thorax may bruise or even rupture the heart without injuring overlying soft tissue or bone. Signs, symptoms, and electrocardiographic changes produced by the contusion are similar to those of myocardial infarction. Myocardial contusions are often produced by open-heart massage and can also be produced by closed-heart massage. The investigator must inform himself concerning the therapy applied to hospitalized patients in order to sort out the various possible causes of cardiac contusions.

Lacerations are tears in tissue due to direct blows by a blunt instrument, crushing, sudden alterations of internal pressure, torsion, and stretching. Internal lacerations are greater threats to life than those on the skin, but their location and extent are not apparent on external examination; in fact, external wounds may be minor even when there is extensive crushing of the internal organs.

The external lacerations of skin are two general types. The direct blow on tissue over a bony prominence will crush the tissues, producing irregular wounds with badly damaged borders. Tiny threads of tissue may bridge these wounds. Hemorrhage is often slight because of sealing of blood vessels by the crushing. One margin may be severely crushed while the other is sharp, indicating obliquity of the blow. The pattern of the object may remain. Injury to bone and deeper structures should be suspected. The other type is a true tear due to twisting or stretching of tissues. The borders are irregular, but the edges are much sharper than those caused by a direct blow. These wounds can cause death by hemorrhage. Both types can result from the same traumatic episode, as is frequently the case in automobile injuries.

Fractures and dislocations are produced by the same forces that produce contusions and lacerations. They need not appear at the same site but often do. Most are recognized by abnormal mobility and posture of the injured area. The excessive mobility of the flaccid neck after death often leads the medical examiner to make an erroneous diagnosis of fracture dislocation of cervical vertebra. This is not a very common injury; it is seen as a result of automobile collisions, falls from high places, or diving accidents. Unless the deformity is great, recognition after death is best done at autopsy. This type of fracture compresses or lacerates the spinal cord and will cause almost instantaneous death or paralysis. Fractures of the skull are considered elsewhere. Numerous fractures of ribs may cause such flaccidity of the thorax that respiratory movements are ineffective. The broken ribs may lacerate pleura, lungs, and heart. Fractures of bones are often associated with severe, soft-tissue injuries and hemorrhage.

The pathologist will often find lipidic emboli in lungs, brain, and kidneys following fractures. This is a much feared complication, but although common to minor degrees, it is rarely the cause of death. The presence of fat emboli is not conclusive evidence of trauma; they are present in small numbers in persons who have not been injured prior to death (1).

REFERENCES

1. Hendrix, R. C., and Fox, J. E.: Relation of obesity and abnormalities of lipid metabolism to lipid embolization of lungs. Am J Clin Pathol, 41:55-60, 1964.

Chapter 14

INJURY BY THERMAL, ELECTRICAL, AND IONIZING ENERGY

THERMAL INJURY

Persons trapped in conflagrations may be partially cremated so that recognition is impossible. This type of burning can occur with fires in a building, wrecked aircraft, and (rarely) highway traffic collisions. The tragedy of the fire in the ship Noronic in Toronto and the masterful identification of the cremated victims will be long remembered (1).

The medical examiner when faced with a partly cremated body must decide, among other things, whether the person was alive or dead when first exposed to the fire. This particular determination is simple; the dead body will not absorb carbon monoxide. The living body inhaling products of combustion will accumulate detectable amounts of carbon monoxide. Aspiration of smoke will cause deposition of carbon particles in the air passages. Actual thermal injury of the airway below the vocal cords does not occur during life. The cremated body should be examined by x-ray if necessary for injuries inconsistent with those produced by fire and to locate foreign bodies. Long bones and the skull can explode due to internal pressures. This type of damage must be distinguished from antemortem trauma which it may simulate closely. Foreign bodies are of particular interest as possible injurious agents and as items of identification. Splitting of skin in a rather sharp pattern may produce a lesion that must be distinguished from antemortem laceration.

Heat coagulates protein and produces shrinkage of muscles and other tissues. This process causes the peculiar posture of the charred body often called the "pugilistic" attitude. The arms are flexed in front of the body; hips and knees are usually flexed also. This posture does not reflect any premortem activity. It occurs in all bodies exposed to intense heat.

Pathologists should be aware that fluids, including blood, are often "cooked" out of the tissues and that this process may simulate subdural hematomas or hemothorax.

Many deaths associated with conflagrations will be due to asphyxia or carbon monoxide intoxication rather than to heat, and bodies may be found without evidence of thermal injury. Carbon monoxide poisoning and other prolonged anoxic states can cause formation of cutaneous blisters which should not be confused with heat effect.

Scalding by hot fluids or gases is seldom immediately fatal except in connection with a major industrial accident. A scald that is less than total can often be recognized long after the injury by the pattern made by rivulets of hot fluid coursing over the body. Scalds are not as destructive to tissues as is open flame, but a large scald will present the same risk of complications.

Persons who survive the immediate incident may die within a few days due to massive burn, hypovolemic shock, or severe chemical laryngotracheobronchitis and pneumonitis, or within weeks or months because of septicemia or bacterial pneumonitis. Renal failure is a possible complication during the first few days to weeks after a severe burn. The long series of reconstructive surgical procedure that is often necessary has its own threats to life. DEATHS DUE TO THE COMPLICATIONS OF VIOLENCE MUST BE INVESTIGATED BY THE MEDICAL EXAMINER (IN MOST JURISDICTIONS) REGARDLESS OF THE LENGTH OF SURVIVAL.

Burning is not a common form of suicide, but it is receiving much publicity at present. Some people, not always oriental fanatics, make a public spectacle of their deaths; others destroy themselves in private. The comments which have been made in the chapter on suicide are relevant here. Intentional homicide with the deliberate use of heat is rare; this form of injury may be directed against children who can be deliberately scalded. Deaths occurring in fires which have been deliberately set are classified as homicides. The vast majority of burns and deaths due to burns are accidental.

Sunburn, although it can be serious, seldom presents a

medicolegal problem. A related oddity, which might contribute to medicolegal investigation on a rare occasion, is that a recently dead body can tan when exposed to bright sunlight (1) (Fig. 20). This change is most apparent in persons with moderately dark complexions.

ELECTRICAL INJURY

Electrical energy can disrupt the function of the conduction system of the heart or the electrochemical processes of the central nervous system. The former causes asystole or arrhythmia incompatible with life, and the latter produces respiratory paralysis. First aid with rapid institution of cardiac and respiratory resuscitative measures can save lives in these conditions. There

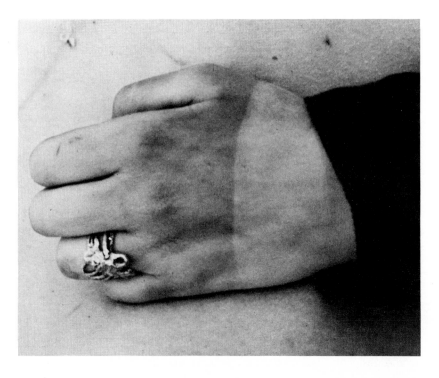

Figure 20. Postmortem hyperpigmentation due to sunlight. The individually hand-crafted ring is an important clue to identity.

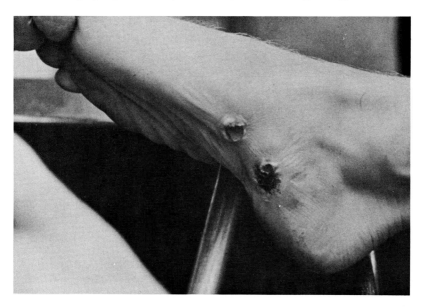

Figure 21. Electrical burns. Decedent touched an electrical transmission wire with a metal pole. Hands and feet were burned.

may be no morphologic evidence of electrocution. The only possible evidence would be at the points of contact of the skin. Dry skin has high resistance to the passage of electric current; heat is developed, and rather characteristic deep, dry burns are produced (Fig. 21). If the skin was wet, or sweaty, at the time of contact, resistance may have been too low to allow for production of heat. Electrocution in a bathtub is a not-uncommon accident that leaves no mark. High-voltage current that is used in transmission lines almost always causes severe burns. The 110-volt current in the usual household circuits can be lethal if the person is in contact with a source of current and a good ground.

Most electrical deaths are accidental; they may occur in the course of employment and are of interest to workmen's compensation commissions. The source of the electrical energy should be apparent, but occasionally it is obscure, and real service can be rendered and lives saved in the future if the recognition of death by electrocution can point to the responsible defective equipment. Domestic accidents are not common but must be considered when death cannot be explained otherwise. Children and pets are sometimes killed by chewing on electrical wiring.

Suicide has been accomplished by means of ordinary household electricity. Some elaborate devices have been prepared for this purpose. Homicide, particularly in infants, has been reported.

Lightning is a very powerful electrical discharge. Its actions are extremely erratic. A person may survive even though most of his clothing is destroyed or he may be killed with little evidence of injury. One or more members of a goup can be killed while others with apparently equal exposure will survive. There may be no marks on the body, there may be a tree-like design of erythema on the skin, there may be small burns adjacent to metal buckles or buttons, or there may be severe incineration. The investigator is rarely faced with a diagnostic problem.

A good many fires are started by electricity; either natural or manmade electricity can cause fires in the home or in the forests. The damage to tissue of humans exposed to the fires is thermal.

EXPOSURE TO COLD

No one "freezes to death" in the literal sense, because death will occur at body temperatures much above the freezing point of body fluids. It is best to consider these deaths as hypothermic, because they occur under circumstances that do not involve freezing temperatures. Elderly persons with mental confusion may wander away from home or institution in inclement weather and die of exposure. Infants are prone to injury of this type and may die when abandoned in exposed places. Extremes of cold will endanger even healthy persons who do not have adequate protection, and continued exposure to very low temperatures will produce literal freezing.

The circumstances in which a body is found are more helpful in recognizing hypothermia than are other aspects of the investigation. These persons will not be cyanotic, rather the skin color will be redder than normal and may cause suspicion of carbon monoxide poisoning. The redness is often blotchy, and chemical studies are negative. All postmortem changes are delayed as long as low temperature of the body is maintained.

Since these bodies are often found in unusual places, and since the deaths are unexplained, careful study is necessary to eliminate the possibility of injury or natural disease. Autopsy will usually be necessary for these reasons.

IONIZING RADIATION

The widespread use of sources of ionizing radiation in medicine, scientific research, and industry is a potential source of fatal injury. The statutes of some states list deaths due to ionizing radiation specifically as requiring investigation by the medical examiner. The medicolegal investigator is seldom faced with a diagnostic dilemma in this area. The type of radiation injury that produces sudden deaths is so catastrophic that no question as to the nature of the problem exists (3). Delayed deaths or deaths related to chronic exposure are usually so well documented medically that there is no diagnostic problem. This is a form of trauma, however, and it is probable that the medical examiner should be notified. The source of irradiation should be identified as protection to others if that has not already been accomplished.

REFERENCES

1. Brown, T. C., Delaney, R. J., and Robinson, W. L.: Medical identification in the Noronic disaster. JAMA, 148:621, 1952.
2. Meirowsky, E.: Uber pigmentbilding in vom Korper losgeloster haut. Frankfurter Ztschr Pathol, 2:438-448, 1909.
3. Liebow, A. A., Warren, S., and Delousey, E.: Pathology of atom bomb casualities. Am J Pathol, 25:853, 1949.

Chapter 15

DROWNING

DROWNING is a common form of accidental death. Water sports are popular and mishaps frequent. Drowning is used as a method of suicide often accompanied by a jump from a high place. As a means of homicide, drowning received some publicity because of gangland executions in the Prohibition era, and it is still encountered on occasion. Disposal of dead bodies in water is also attempted; some of these are attempts to conceal a body, some are attempts to disguise other forms of death.

Accidental drowning related to water sports is usually witnessed. The witnesses often give a story of unsuccessful attempts at rescue and resuscitation. The bodies will be dressed in appropriate attire; any inappropriateness of dress should raise suspicion of other than accidental means of death. The medical examiner should also be prepared to ask searching questions concerning the death of a good swimmer under circumstances that are not markedly hazardous. What were the circumstances? Who was with the deceased at the time? What was his state of health? What was his level of intoxication? Was he attempting some form of endurance test?

The body recovered from water after a period of immersion of no more than a few hours length will show few external signs of the cause of death. There may be rather voluminous stiff white froth at the mouth and nares (Fig. 22). The skin and mucous membranes may be pinker than normal if the water was cold, and cutis anserina may be prominent. Except for the froth, which is a manifestation of rapidly developing pulmonary edema, these are postmortem changes. None is diagnostic. Prolonged submersion following drowning produces changes that do not differ from prolonged submersion following death from any cause. The skin of hands or feet will become white and wrinkled. Body temperature will rapidly reach that of the water. If that temperature is high,

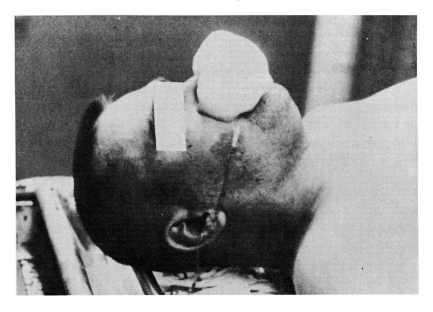

Figure 22. Drowning. The froth may not develop in some very rapid deaths by drowning.

putrefaction will be rapid and the gases produced will cause the body to float in a few days. This process is slower in colder waters and may not occur at all when the temperature is very low. Scavenger fish and turtles can hasten destruction of the body.

Serious problems arise when a body is found in water, and there is no indication of the events that caused it to be there and no information concerning the length of time that it has been there. Identification will be the first problem to be solved. The techniques of identification have been considered in Chapter 4. Once identification has been made, time of disappearance can be determined, and the destination and plans of the deceased may be discovered. Knowledge of plans for a fishing or hunting trip, combined with appropriate equipment on or near the body, will aid in the final decision.

Special note should be made of restraints which might have impaired the person's ability to save himself. The possibility that the restraints, if present, were of such nature that they could not have been applied by the victim must be considered. External evidence of violence other than drowning should be sought.

Any found body, whether in water or not, should be subjected to autopsy unless antecedent events are exceptionally well documented. The necessity for autopsy increases with advanced deterioration. No body is too deteriorated for an autopsy, although the task may be an unpleasant one. The morphologic criteria for drowning are not entirely conclusive. The external appearance of the recently drowned body has been described. Internally there will be pulmonary congestion, massive pulmonary edema, and the nonspecific evidences of anoxia. The deceased may have ingested large amounts of water. These observations will be confirmed microscopically, and, in addition, bits of debris or plankton from natural waters will be present in alveoli. With these findings and without evidence of trauma or significant natural disease, the diagnosis of death by drowning can be made with some degree of confidence. Aspiration of water does not always occur. Therefore, the absence of particulate matter in the air passages does not eliminate the possibility of drowning, although the degree of certainty is reduced.

Because of this lack of certainty and because many bodies removed from water are traumatized or badly deteriorated, the need for definite tests has been recognized. The chloride test is based on the fact that there will be a change in electrolytes in the pulmonary capillaries exposed to water in the alveoli. If the water is fresh (and unpolluted), chlorides will dialize from the blood, and a sample removed from the left side of the heart will have a lower chloride concentration than one from the right. If the drowning is in ocean water, the blood in the pulmonary capillaries will pick up chlorides (and other electrolytes) with a reversal of the analytic values. If the drowning has been in tidal and brackish rivers, no conclusions can be drawn. The rapid alteration of intracellular and extracellular electrolytes after death so limits the value of this method that it is seldom used. The specific gravity test is based on similar principles and is subject to the same uncontrolled variables. It is not popular at the present time.

The diatom test was developed in Europe. It was observed that fine particles aspirated into the lung could enter the blood stream and be carried to distant parts of the body. The silicaceous shells of the diatoms (minute algea found in large numbers in most natural waters) are readily recognizable. Tissues such as bone, liver, and spleen were digested and the resulting fluid was filtered or centrifuged and examined for diatoms. Algae were found in the tissues of victims of drowning, and there was some correlation between the number and kind in tissues and in the water. Unfortunately, diatoms are so very numerous and widely distributed in drinking water (both treated and untreated) and in dust and have such a wide industrial use (including filtration of municipal water supplies) that their presence is not an entirely reliable indication of death by drowning. In difficult cases, the presence or absence of these algae, when added to other infomation, will add a degree of confidence to one's decision. This seems to be one of the best tests available. The entire subject has been reviewed recently by Timperman (1).

The presence of debris and plankton from natural waters in the peripheral portions of the lung is strong presumptive evidence that the subject was alive when he entered the water. The significance of this finding has been attacked on experimental and theoretical grounds, but experience has demonstrated that it is just as useful as many of the more complicated tests.

When investigating the unexplained drowning, the medical examiner must always consider the possibility that the individual was rendered unconscious by blows or drugs and placed in the water or was physically forced in the water. Head trauma which is severe enough to produce unconsciousness will often produce subgaleal hemorrhage even though no bruise is visible on the surface of the scalp. Once chemical and physical trauma and natural disease have been ruled out, the death may be attributed to drowning; nonmedical evidence would be needed to determine the cause of drowning.

Bizarre situations are encountered at every turn in medicolegal investigation, and investigation of drownings is no exception. Persons are found apparently drowned in situations which they should have been able to avoid or from which they should have been able to escape. Healthy individuals do not drown inadvertently in bathtubs or in puddles in a rutted road, for example. Other factors must exist and should be found.

REFERENCES

1. Timperman, J.: Medicolegal problem in death by drowning. Its diagnosis by the diatom method. A study based on investigation carried out in Ghent over a period of 10 years. J Forensic Med, 16:45-75, 1969.

Chapter 16

MECHANICAL ASPHYXIA

HANGING

Hanging is a very common method of suicide; accidental hanging is not rare. Homicidal hanging is extremely unusual, but postmortem hanging may be used to obscure other causes of death.

The professional hangman arranges a fall which is stopped suddenly by a noose and a rope. Fracture dislocation of the cervical vertebra with transection of spinal cord are produced, and death is instantaneous. Amateur hanging is not so arranged, and death is due to constriction of arteries, veins, and airways. The vascular obstruction is probably most important and certainly is responsible for the very rapid loss of consciousness that occurs. Full suspension is not necessary for a fatal outcome. Partial suspension from a door knob can put enough weight on the ligature to constrict vessels and possibly the airway. The first person to find the body in a hanging or semi-hanging position will often release the ligature and attempt resuscitation or may attempt to conceal the true nature of the death. The ligature will almost always leave a mark around the neck; subcutaneous adipose tissue will be crushed, and the freed lipid will soak into the dermis and produce a parchment-like appearance and texture (Fig. 23). This appearance is enhanced by prolonged pressure and by drying. Hemorrhages are usually present in the deeper soft tissues of the neck. Hyoid bone and thyroid cartilages may or may not be fractured, depending upon the position of the ligature. The mark made by the ligature on the neck will demonstrate some of the characteristics of the material used (Fig. 23). The braiding of the rope, the weave of the fabric, or the web marks on the strap may be impressed on the skin, and possibly the cross-sectional shape may be evident. The arrangement of the ligature and number of

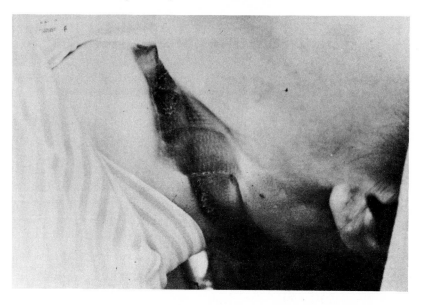

Figure 23. Hanging. The parchment-like change in skin, the fabric pattern of the ligature, and the type of knot are apparent.

loops will be apparent, and the weight-bearing loop will leave a somewhat elliptical mark directed toward the point of suspension (Fig. 24). On occasion, a very broad, soft fabric such as a bath towel may be used for ligature and may produce very faint marks on the neck.

Since hanging causes vascular constriction, a marked congestion of the tissue above the ligature will often be found. This congestion will be independent of the type of ligature, and its localization to the head, the sharp border, and circumferential uniformity will help distinguish from the congestion which often develops with a myocardial infarct or the hypostasis developing in a body in head-down position.

Ideally, evidence of suicidal hanging will consist of the changes in the body described above, a ligature, and an accessible object from which the body can be completely or partly suspended. If the hands or feet are bound (and suicides may do this) the possibility of self-application must exist. As in all suicides, one

INDEX